Limitless Health

A Simple Guide to Reaching Your Health Goals and Making Better Choices in the Moment

Tammy Fogarty, Ph.D., RD

Copyright © 2023 Tammy Fogarty

All rights reserved. No part of this book may be reproduced in any form without permission from the author or publisher, except as permitted by U.S. copyright law.

To request permission, contact Tammy Fogarty at tammy@tammyfogarty.com

Photography and Cover Design by Erika Hanchar-Walker
Edited by Caroline Barnhill

ISBN: 979-8-9893118-0-4
Printed in the United States of America
First edition

Published by Tammy Fogarty
www.tammyfogarty.com

Table of Contents

DEDICATION 5
DISCLAIMER 7
WELCOME 9
INTRODUCTION 11
DAY 1: BECOME YOUR DEFINITION OF HEALTHY 23
DAY 2: DIETS SUCK 29
DAY 3: I LOVE CARBS 37
DAY 4: THE SKINNY ON FATS 49
DAY 5: PROTEIN: IT'S SO MUCH MORE THAN BUILDING MUSCLES 55
DAY 6: SHHHH... YOUR BODY IS TRYING TO TELL YOU SOMETHING 63
DAY 7: PROACTIVE, NOT REACTIVE 71
DAY 8: DO WHAT YOU LOVE 79
DAY 9: PRIORITIZE PHYSICAL ACTIVITY 89
DAY 10: SET A GOAL. OR DON'T. CHOOSE WHAT WORKS FOR YOU. 97
DAY 11: OVERCOME CHALLENGES 105
DAY 12: RETHINK YOUR DRINK 115
DAY 13: OUT OF SIGHT, OUT OF MIND 121
DAY 14: GO TO BED 127
DAY 15: HEY, YOUR GUT IS LEAKING 137
DAY 16: YOU ARE ONE BITE AWAY FROM A GOOD MOOD 147
DAY 17: HAVE A PLAN 157
DAY 18: DON'T BREAK THE BANK 165
DAY 19: WINNING THE BATTLE AGAINST OVERINDULGENCE ... 173
DAY 20: DATE NIGHT 181

DAY 21: CREATE THE LIFE YOU WANT TO LIVE 187
ACKNOWLEDGMENTS 193
ABOUT THE AUTHOR 195

Dedication

To my mom, who taught me to embrace life's challenges with strength and grace. May this book honor the legacy you left behind and the profound impact you had on my life.

Forever in my thoughts, forever in my heart.

Disclaimer

The information provided in this nutrition book is for general informational purposes only and should not be considered medical advice. It is not intended to diagnose, treat, cure, or prevent any medical condition. Always consult with a qualified healthcare professional before making any changes to your diet, exercise routine, or lifestyle.

The content of this book is based on the author's research, personal experiences, and knowledge of nutrition and health up to the publication date. However, individual nutritional needs and health conditions can vary widely. What works for one person may not work for another, and what is suitable for some may not be suitable for others.

Any recommendations, suggestions, or guidelines provided in this book should not be interpreted as a substitute for medical advice, diagnosis, or treatment. Readers should seek the advice of a qualified healthcare provider with any questions or concerns they may have regarding their health.

The author, publisher, and any other parties involved in the creation and distribution of this book disclaim any liability for any adverse effects or consequences resulting from the use of the information provided. Readers should use their own discretion and judgment when applying any information from this book to their personal health and wellness journey.

Always remember that medical knowledge is constantly evolving, and new research may emerge that could impact the information provided in this book. It is important to stay informed about the latest developments in nutrition and healthcare and to consult with qualified professionals when making decisions about your health.

In summary, while this book aims to provide useful and accurate information about nutrition, readers should always prioritize their health and safety by consulting with medical professionals and registered dietitians before making any significant changes to their diet or lifestyle.

Welcome

Congratulations on investing in your health and being brave enough to try something new. This book is designed to help you identify health goals that truly matter and to provide clear strategies to create long-term healthy habits. As we move through stages of life, our health goals and priorities will change. The strategies in this book can be applied to men and women at any time throughout the stages of life. Take what works for you and backburner items that don't currently resonate with you. I encourage you to utilize the strategies of this book to create a custom-designed plan to achieve your goals and desires.

Introduction

Have you ever felt overwhelmed by the endless array of diets and conflicting nutritional advice?

Do you find yourself wondering if there's a better way to improve your health?

What if the secret to a healthier, happier life is not just what you eat but how you understand and approach nutrition, exercise, sleep, and stress?

In the hustle and bustle of our modern lives, we often forget that the most powerful medicine we have is found not in a pill bottle, but within the choices you make every day. Did you know that it's possible to alter your behaviors, such as the foods you eat and ways to reduce stress, and still feel fulfilled, accomplished, and motivated to do more?

Of course, you do (or plan to). That's why you are reading this book. At some point, you have tried a lifestyle change and have felt great about it. But now you want more, if you can get over that tiny problem of *where, when, and how to start!* You want to lose weight; you plan to exercise more; you hate feeling stressed. You want to fix everything but are overwhelmed and unsure where to begin. Add to it the anxiety and frustrations you feel and the voice in your head saying, *I should have accomplished so much more by now.*

This scenario is common, and I have helped many people in the same situation as you. They want to get healthy and have big plans to make changes. But change is not easy, and with it comes the fear of what lies ahead.

That's why I wrote this book and created online nutrition classes: to give you a roadmap to find clarity, take action, and build momentum to finally achieve your health goals and feel good about yourself. Over the years, my clients have struggled with at least one of these three core issues:

1. You can't find the time.
    - *I want to get healthy but struggle to find the time to do anything for myself. Between work and the kids, I rarely have a moment to myself. How do I juggle all my obligations and still have time to eat healthy and hit the gym?*

2. You are unsure what approach will work best.
    - *I am unsure what to do: lift weights, do cardio, eat a high-fat diet, or run a marathon. It's all so overwhelming. How do I know what will work for me?*

3. You keep trying but are not seeing results.
    - *I have tried every diet in the book, I eat healthy, but I still cannot lose weight. I get so frustrated that I just give up and eat what I love instead. None of these diets work anyway.*

If you struggle with any of these issues, trust that you are not alone and are in the right place. You will learn different techniques to achieve your goals and effectively strategize your day to achieve small wins constantly. But before I move on, I want to ensure we are on the same page.

This book is not a quick-fix diet or instructions on how to gain 6-pack abs. And you need to understand that change is not easy. In fact, it may be the most challenging thing that you do. The goal is to be open-minded, try new things, and strive to be your best. Nothing comes easily, and I want you to aim for daily progress over perfection.

If you choose to continue reading (I sure hope you do), get ready to work hard, throw your ego and excuses out the window, and be prepared to get real with yourself. You will dig deep to find what is important to you, have clarity about the goals that suit you, and be motivated to push through even when you feel like giving up. Because your health is important to you. You want to live a youthful existence. You want to live a life free of disease. **You want limitless health.**

Yes! You are ready. Be ready for some major wins, but also be ready for disappointment. Remember, nothing in life comes easy. But we have already established that you are here to do the work and are ready for change. And the plan I have laid out for you allows you to apply a new, healthy strategy daily – in 10 minutes or less. Do you have 10 minutes per day to do something good for yourself? I believe you do.

Go big or go home does not apply here. Instead, slow and steady wins the race. So, be patient with yourself. Be kind but also challenge yourself. Welcome what is unfamiliar and be open-minded to try new things.

While there are no guarantees that my book will work for you, there are ways to set yourself up for the best chance of success. You've got to be honest with yourself about your mindset, skills, strengths, and limitations. Prove to yourself that you can accomplish anything you set your mind to.

There are theories and practices to help you make behavioral changes that lead to smart choices and build momentum to continue this journey. That's exactly what this book is designed to help you achieve.

As you implement these practices, the goal is to gain clarity and self-awareness and build up small wins and confidence as you make progress. You can't successfully achieve your health goal just by reading and learning about it; you must apply what you have learned by choosing the Achievable Actions at the end of each chapter – or in the case of this book, each day.

Before I share all the amazing things you will gain from reading this book, I want to share how nutrition changed my life.

About Me

As a child, I was carefree, happy, and silly. My days centered around riding my bike after school, playing with dolls, and blissfully eating junk food. A simple, fun life doing what kids love. It was me and my mom for most of my childhood and teen years. She was a single parent and the most fantastic mother anyone could ask for. She is the reason I was so happy and carefree.

But my childhood wasn't all fun and games. My simple childhood turned into me being a caregiver when I was eight years old. My mom was diagnosed with breast cancer in her early thirties. I was in third grade when she began a 14-year battle that included chemotherapy, radiation, and surgery to remove her breasts. I helped by doing laundry, cleaning, and preparing dinner. I hated making dinner. But, little did I know at the time, those dinners would mean so much more than just another chore.

Our lives had several ups and downs during my mom's 14-year battle with breast cancer. The greatest challenge was the unpredictable disease my mom was fighting. She went into remission for some time; however, the cancer would return and spread to her bones, causing great pain and discomfort. Thankfully, she always remained positive. She was unwaveringly positive and confident, even when her doctors informed us that few options remained and that time was of the essence. However, the news did not deter my mom from beating cancer, and shortly after, we received a book from my cousin titled *A Cancer Battle Plan* by Ann Frohm. Within the pages of this book, we learned about a heroic woman who took control of her health with unconventional treatments, including food.

FOOD? Yes, *food*. In our house, we didn't think much about *what* we ate. Instead, we ate what we loved, like pizza, pasta, and hot dogs. Hot dogs were my all-time favorite and became a staple in my diet. Like every other household, the house always had soda, ice cream, cereal, white bread, and pastries. But as I started reading more about the healing potential of nutrients, I realized we had an opportunity to use food in a medicinal way to help my mom fight the most challenging fight of her life. And it was simple. We just had to eat healthy foods. And this is how dinner came to mean so much to me. At the end of each day, we prepared simple, nutritious meals to give my mom the nourishment her body needed to fight the good fight. And much to our surprise, she started feeling better. Her energy was restored, she was happy, she started dating, and she felt good. Most importantly, her health improved, and she could take small breaks from treatment. This simple approach to health led to significant changes, and it all started with what we put on our dinner plates.

So, what was so special about dinner? Dinner became a time to unwind from the day, nourish our bodies with healthy foods, and, most importantly, spend quality time with each other. We learned so much about *what* was in our foods and how the "junky" food we loved, including my beloved hot dog, could have contributed to my mom being diagnosed with breast cancer. For the first time, we realized that foods have a purpose and that each nutrient has a unique role in supporting the immune system. All we had to do was make healthy choices. It was simple. Coincidentally, Mom's tumor markers decreased after we changed our diet, and she was so close to being in remission again.

It was almost too simple. *But could it be this easy?* For us, making these changes meant that my mom's immune system and her body would become stronger. Changing how we ate meant something and became the most important thing that we *had* to do. We shifted our typical diets from fast foods to nourishing meals, *and it was easy.* Each meal had a purpose and was loaded with nutrients. We ate fruit, vegetables, fish, and whole grains. And we felt amazing!

Dinners with Mom became a time to educate ourselves, laugh, cry, and make decisions, including my decision to study nutrition. I saw how this simple change affected us, and I was hungry to learn more. I wanted to share with others how the course of my Mom's battle with cancer changed after nutrition became a priority. We were on a *non-processed* sugar high!

But this journey had more twists and turns in store for us.

We felt good and had good intentions to continue our newfound lifestyle. However, the novelty eventually disappeared, as with most "new" things. The novelty of our new, simple, healthy lifestyle wore off, and old habits and the familiar comforts of our favorite foods crept back into our routine. Life continued, as it always does.

My mom continued working two jobs, sometimes three, to support us. I was in college, studying to be a nutritionist, so I had to work at night, and dinners with Mom became less frequent. Despite studying nutrition, convenience foods and drive-thru fast-food restaurants felt necessary after long days.

Unfortunately, my mom started to feel less energetic and less motivated. She was tired and frail, and her eyes confirmed what we were afraid to say aloud. We no longer received glowing results from her doctor. The cancer continued to spread. This time, they found a spot on her head, so radiation was ordered, resulting in the loss of vision in one eye. Then, a PET scan found spots on her lungs, and she required oxygen. The nurses at the hospital got to know my mom since blood transfusions became routine. Her favorite nurse, Hal, was the only person she trusted to place the IV. His eyes, too, confirmed the words we were so afraid to speak.

My mom said her final word on March 4, 2000, "No." She wasn't ready to go. After all, she was only 47 years old. F*ing cancer won. She repeated the word "NO" as she took her last breath. My mom was a strong, resilient woman her entire life. And she left this world fighting. Fighting for her life, fighting for me, and for the life she wouldn't get to live.

I learned so much from my mom. Most importantly, she taught me to stand on my own two feet and not depend on others. She would say that I had to find my way and be able to take care of myself. And I achieved that goal, but I also wanted to take care of others and help individuals fighting any battle with a disease. Nutrition is powerful. I saw its powers firsthand with my mom. But it's not just nutrition; there are several factors we must consider to achieve wellness.

After Mom passed, I finished my bachelor's degree in Dietetics and Nutrition and earned a master's and a Ph.D. in Nutrition. My career as a dietitian-nutritionist began in the hospital setting and evolved into higher education. My private practice provides medical nutrition therapy to those who choose an integrative healthcare approach. I had the privilege of sharing my knowledge with a group of breast cancer survivors who participated in my 6-week nutrition and yoga intervention to improve quality of life as my Ph.D. dissertation. Everything I'd worked so hard for came to fruition. There is always a silver lining with any disease, and Mom's illness and her struggles with breast cancer helped shape the person I am today.

I miss our dinners. I miss our laughs, our cries, and our fight for wellness. I miss my mom terribly. As horrible as that journey was, it has led me here to you. And I am writing this book to share with you all I have learned along the way. I am the same age today as my mom was when she passed. Being healthy has become my mission, and I absolutely intend to scream what I know from the rooftops. The most important lessons I have learned thus far are:

- Being healthy doesn't have to be complicated.
- Staying healthy doesn't have to be a chore.
- Small changes cause significant results.
- There is no reason to complicate your life.
- Stop making excuses. You are in control of your life.

I wrote this book to demonstrate how small changes can be impactful. Living a healthy life is easy. Unfortunately, we tend to associate change with hardship. It means moving away from what we are comfortable with and transitioning into a space that makes us uncomfortable. We crave comfort even if it means sacrificing our health.

It's safe to assume that you no longer want to sacrifice your health and you are looking for guidance to move you in a new direction. But, to do so, you have to make changes. I understand the challenges that come with change, so I am going to make it as simple as possible for you.

My goal is that you will try something new daily. Each day, you have one mission. Your mission is to pick at least one achievable action, found at the end of each chapter. I encourage you to do all of them, but you must choose at least one. The next day, you will choose another action, while continuing to do the action you chose the day before. Over the next twenty-one days, you will have tried twenty-one new actions that will enhance your well-being. As you repeatedly do these actions daily, they will eventually become a *habit*. At the end of this book, you will have mastered strategies that can transcend your life and allow you to conquer any goal. You are one bite away from living a happy life.

What you will get out of this book

In this book, you will discover what you need to know to understand the role of food and nutrients and why choosing or limiting certain foods is important. Most importantly, you will know what to do to get started today. The best part is that you can achieve this without sacrificing the foods you love with complicated fad diets and restrictive meal plans. The first step is to determine what it means to you to be healthy. This step is crucial to understanding your motivations and ensuring you're clear and focused on your health goals.

Next, you will set aside time each day to read one chapter. But rather than chapters, the book includes 21 days of reading and is designed to give you one to three strategies for that day. I have arranged the days in a sequence that makes sense to me and has helped numerous clients achieve their goals. However, you can choose which day to read based on your health goal(s).

Along the way, I will challenge you to be honest with yourself, answer tough questions, and make clear decisions. Most importantly, you will execute a plan of action. At the end of each day, you will see a summary and list of Achievable Actions. Remember that you have a choice in every moment. Take that moment to decide your plan of action for the day. You will also receive access to additional resources at www.tammyfogarty.com to help you dig deeper, strategize, and track your progress.

What you won't get out of this book

This book is not a diet, a meal plan, or rules to follow. I do not provide weekly grocery lists or recommend dietary restrictions. This book does not promise you will lose weight or run a marathon; that is up to you to decide. You must also determine the strategies that work for you. Lastly, this book does not provide medical advice or recommendations to use or discontinue medications, specific supplements, or diet pills.

Instead, this book will provide information and strategies to empower you to make informed decisions, which will lead to impactful choices that improve your health and well-being.

Are you ready to unleash your limitless potential to achieve your ultimate health and wellness goal?

The definition of a limit is a *boundary* or *end*. To be a *limitless person* means to be someone *without end, limit, or boundary* (Oxford Languages, n.d.). In a sense, limitless is realizing and embracing our inner superhero, and we all have one. A person who lives without limits can create the life they want to live. No limits mean exactly that: **no limits.** What would it feel like to be limitless?

But to be limitless, we need to live without limitations. Limitations can be related to physical abilities, overall health, and dietary limitations. Right now, you may have physical restrictions that limit your ability to exercise. For example, do you suffer from back or knee pain that makes physical activities impossible? Certain health conditions create limitations that hinder the ability to travel, eat certain foods, and exercise. Individuals with diabetes must ensure they have all their medications when they travel and need to closely monitor what they eat or suffer the consequences of high or low blood sugar. In addition, dietary restrictions due to lifestyle choices may limit specific foods and create nutrient deficiencies. What limitations do you suffer from?

Can you imagine what your life could look like if you had no limitations?

Would you be free of pain?

Free to eat without feeling bloated?

Free from stress?

Free to live a simple, healthy life?

Free to live without limits?

Limitless health refers to the ability to live a healthy life without the limitations of disease, stress, and physical inabilities. If you had no limitations, *who* would you be?

- If you did not have physical limitations, could you be a runner?
- If you did not battle with fatigue, could you be a motivator?
- If you did not have dietary restrictions, could you be healthy?
- If you did not follow a strict diet, could you be carefree?

There is no such thing as eternal health, although that would be awesome. Some things are completely out of our control, such as age, gender, and race. However, we can control many factors that affect health, such as what we eat, how much we eat, how we handle stress, and how physically active we are. These factors are the leading causes of health or disease. If we live a healthy life, we can also live a life with unlimited potential. What would your life look like?

This book is not an instruction manual on how to lose weight or get a perfectly sculpted body. This book is a guide to empower you to make decisions that will affect your ability to lose weight, reduce stress, become more physically active, and live up to your limitless potential. We are faced with daily choices: pick the French fries or a side salad, get up or hit snooze, go for a jog or sink into the couch. Today, you have chosen to read this book. And for the next 21 days, you will receive advice and recommendations backed by scientific research. You will also receive actionable tools designed to help you become limitless. Each day, you choose which strategies to implement so that you are one step closer to meeting your health goals.

As a registered dietitian and licensed nutritionist, I have devoted my life to helping individuals realize their potential to make healthy behavioral changes. I provide my clients with individual plans to reach their goals through nutrition counseling. I cannot provide you with an individual nutrition plan, but I can provide you with the tools and effective strategies that have worked with my clients. While I don't pretend to have all the answers, I aim to help you find yours.

I know that time is a factor that affects the choices we make. And, since we are all busy and short on time, I have designed this book so that you can learn and apply a new approach to achieving health and wellness in as little as 10 minutes. Each day, I will present you with choices you can implement that will work for you. Eating healthy is easy. What's difficult is making the decision to do so. Throughout this book, I will provide you with simple choices so you no longer have to make the hard decisions.

The choice is yours. Are you ready to live a simple, healthy life with limitless potential?

Day 1

Become YOUR Definition of Healthy

Welcome to Day 1. Before we start, I would like to explain an essential component of wellness: self-efficacy. Self-efficacy is a person's belief in their ability to complete a task, achieve a goal, and meet challenges head-on. Self-efficiency is the ability to take control of one's life and attain goals that serve a purpose. It is also the *belief in yourself* to make impactful choices that promote health and wellness.

We all set goals for ourselves, but achieving them is not always easy unless you have the know-how and tools to make them happen. I want you to consider this book a guide to achieving self-efficacy. At the end of 21 days, you will have a toolbox full of strategies to attain any goal you set your mind to. The first step towards self-efficacy is to define what being healthy means to you. *What* does healthy look like? *Why* do you want to be healthy? *Who* could you be when you are healthy?

The term *healthy* can refer to several aspects of a person's life. To me, healthy refers to the overall physical, mental, and spiritual wellness that fuels the body and engages the mind-body connection. But there are many aspects of health, and the first thing I want you to do is to identify your definition of health as it stands right now in your life. And keep in mind, the definition of health will evolve as you move through life experiences. Your definition of health today is not set in stone. You may have a completely different mindset at the end of this book.

Throughout the book, I will focus on the role of nutrition in wellness. Still, "healthy" can represent any aspect of wellness, such as physical, emotional, spiritual, or financial wellness. Making the right choices for health and well-being can be challenging, so it is important to take a moment to identify what matters, why you want to make a change, and what your end goal is.

Most importantly, your health goal must be something *you* want to achieve. This is your life, your goal, and your self-efficacy. So, choose something that has meaning to you. As a nutritionist, I have worked with clients who attempted to achieve a goal because their spouse or friend said they should. In the end, they struggled with following through because it was not their goal in the first place. Trust me, you will find every excuse to sabotage the goal; don't waste your time achieving someone else's goal. It is all about YOU.

While achieving a health goal can be challenging, you'll have the resilience and determination you need to succeed when you're doing it for the right reasons. The gratification you feel will guide you past the obstacles and challenges that come your way.

Here's the bottom line of Day One: Determine your definition of health and never work on a goal that does not fulfill you. Each of us is unique, with our custom-sized hopes and dreams and definition of well-being. Rather than letting society's standards dictate the definition of healthy or the goals we must accomplish, I want you to think and dream for yourself. Real success means staying true to yourself and connected to your vision and goals, not society's.

To get started, list the health priorities that mean something to you. Common health goals include:

- Eat healthy
- Lose weight
- Sleep 7 hours per night
- Manage stress
- Be a role model for your kids
- Get organized
- Don't drink so much wine

Okay, that last goal is for me. I love wine and enjoy having a glass, or two, with dinner at night. However, having a glass of wine every night is not the healthiest choice, so I must replace my love for wine with a healthier alternative.

You see, our greatest challenge is letting go of what we enjoy. I enjoy making dinner and sipping on a beautiful cabernet; it relaxes me. But, as a nutritionist, I know that wine provides calories, impairs sleep, decreases motivation, and, most importantly, can increase the risk of breast cancer. My internal struggle is doing what I enjoy vs. doing what is right.

I am sure that you can relate. Deep down, you know how to achieve your health goals. The hardest part is to stop listening to the voice in your head that is making excuses to continue unhealthy behaviors. But remember, you are not reading this book for the easy way out. You are reading this book to find a way to get it done. Jump off that proverbial cliff...rip off the band-aid...stop doing the things that drag you down...stop listening to the voice in your head saying, "You can't do this." Because you can do this. And I promise, by the end of this book, you will look back and realize it wasn't so bad after all. Now, let's get back to that list.

From the list of health goals you created, prioritize your goals. Place a number one next to the goal that means the most to you.

The goal that will fulfill you and make you feel good about yourself. And remember, this is *your* goal and not what anyone else wants you to achieve. Oftentimes, when I work with clients, their end goal is not the goal they came to see me for. Dive deep into your soul, determine what will make you happy, and place a big ol' number 1 next to it. That will be your focus throughout this book.

Continue numbering your list based on priority. As you achieve one goal, move on to the next and then the next. Throughout this book, you will acquire new knowledge and skills so you become *your definition* of healthy.

Summary:

- Self-efficacy is a person's belief in their ability to complete a task, achieve a goal, and meet challenges head-on.
- Self-efficacy is believing in yourself to make informed decisions promoting health and wellness.
- The term "healthy" can refer to several aspects of a person's life and will change as you move through life stages and experiences.

Achievable Actions:

- Make a list of health goals you want to achieve.
- Using that list, prioritize your goals, with number one being the most important goal.

- Write down that goal and place it where you can see it because you will work on achieving this for the next 20 days.

Day 2

Diets Suck

The word "diet" has many different meanings. To me, diet refers to a person's overall eating patterns, such as the foods consumed on a regular basis. It is a pattern of eating, and depending on your food choices, your diet can be healthy, unhealthy, excessive, restrictive, or balanced. For many, the term "diet" is often associated with a plan someone devised that is designed to achieve weight loss. For others, "diet" can mean restricting certain foods; it means going hungry to look a certain way or achieving a specific weight goal. We convince ourselves that restricting certain foods or only eating during certain times of the day will create a physique that, unfortunately, may be too far out of reach. That, my friend, is not the definition of a diet, but rather, it is the definition of a *fad diet*.

A fad diet is a popular dietary pattern known as a quick fix for weight loss. These diets are appealing because they promise immediate results that require little effort. You can identify a fad diet by the following characteristics:

- Promises rapid weight loss
- Exercise is typically not included
- Focuses on one type of food or eliminates a food group
- Is not sustainable long-term

- Is nutritionally inadequate
- Fails to provide health warnings for those with chronic disease
- The person pushing the diet knows nothing about nutrition; hence, it lacks scientific evidence to support claims for weight loss

Fad diets fail to provide an essential component related to weight loss. Remember that fad diets tell you *what* to eat; however, they do not inform you *how* to maintain your current body weight or gym routine. Furthermore, the diet will only take you so far; the rest is up to you. You will regain the weight and possibly more without the necessary tools to sustain weight loss.

Would you start a fad diet knowing it will cause you to gain weight? Research suggests that roughly 80% of people who lose a significant percentage of their body fat will not maintain the weight loss for 12 months. In fact, dieters may regain more than half of what they lost within two years. Fad diets don't work. They never have, and they never will.

Your task for day #2 is simple: ditch the fad diet mindset. I want you to ditch any preconceived notions you have learned, heard about, and plan to try. Instead, I will introduce you to a non-fad diet approach that encourages you to embrace a lifestyle that includes eating healthy foods, exercising, and reducing stress.

The definition of diet is the kind of food that a person habitually eats. Throughout this book, when I refer to your "diet," it is the pattern of food intake you choose to consume, not a weight loss fad. Let's end the negative connotation associated with the term diet. Now that we are clear about diet vs. fad diet, allow me to elaborate on why fad diets don't work.

Here is a common scenario that I have seen too often with my clients. Social media's latest weight loss fad diet promises quick results, so you go all in. All you have to do is restrict your caloric intake by omitting all carbohydrates. By consuming fewer calories, your body will begin burning stored fat for energy, thus causing weight loss. At first, the results are evident, and losing 10-15 pounds is relatively easy. You feel great about yourself and want to show off your leaner curves. You slip into your new skinny jeans, head to your favorite restaurant, and celebrate your accomplishments. Fantastic! You should celebrate.

As the weeks progress, you still feel great but miss the foods you are "not allowed" to eat. So, you may indulge a little in your favorite comfort foods. The gym routine begins to feel too time-consuming; thus, you skip a few days during the week. The voice inside you says, *"What is the harm?"* This is the moment when things go sideways.

You are not sure how to continue this new lifestyle. What should you do when you have food cravings or don't feel like going to the gym? You are gaining weight again, so you return to what feels normal and comfortable. You return to your old way of doing things. Your fad diet has failed you, so you move on to the next one.

Once again, you restrict calories, lose weight, pull those skinny jeans out from the back of your closet, and celebrate. Have you noticed a trend? We celebrate with food. The very thing that you are attempting to control. But the celebration must continue; you welcome comfort foods, and the unwanted pounds return little by little. The skinny jeans are abandoned in the dark corner of your closet, and the quest for a better diet begins. This repetitive cycle is the start of yo-yo-dieting.

Let's take a deeper dive into why fad diets don't work. Fad diets encourage the restriction of specific foods and, ultimately, calories. In the case of yo-yo dieting, the routine of restricting calories for a period of time and then splurging on your favorite foods signals the body to store calories instead of burning calories. The restriction of calories (the fad diet) followed by an influx of calories (the celebration, comfort foods, etc.) prepares your body for the next period of food restriction. At this point, you are training your body to prepare for food deprivation. The body prepares for this period of food restriction by storing more calories than it burns.

Please note that your body has one significant role: *to keep you alive*. The body requires calories from food to produce energy. With fewer calories, we produce less energy for daily activities. As a result, the body will slow down, including your metabolism, heart rate, and respiratory rate, making you feel sluggish. It can also cause a decrease in motivation and disrupt sleep. You may even experience symptoms of anxiety and depression. The more calories your body stores, the less weight you will lose. Weight loss will become more challenging no matter how many diets you try.

Remember that any time you omit an entire food group, such as carbohydrates, you will create a calorie deficit, resulting in weight loss. Restricting calories is effective for short-term weight loss, but omitting a food group will result in more than fewer calories; your diet will be less nutritious, leading to nutrient deficiencies. For example, a high-fat, low-carb diet is typically low in fiber and may cause constipation, hemorrhoids, and other unpleasantries. While fad diets may work in the short term, restrictive diets are challenging to stick to over time. In fact, research on fad diets is limited because few people can maintain a restrictive eating pattern for more than two years. And let's face it, most weight regain occurs within twelve months of starting the diet. Additionally, fad diets are associated with a negative body image and may result in disordered eating.

The other issue is that fad diets tend to demonize certain foods. I am sure we all remember how the poor egg yolk got pulled through the wringer as being the cause of heart disease. Gluten receives a fair amount of negative publicity these days a[s a] punching bag for diet fanatics. Focusing on one nutrient [isn't] the answer. Instead, we must assess the overall quality of o[ur] diet.

Are you ready to ditch the diet mindset? I hope so, because this is your task for today. Instead, I want you to focus on the overall quality of your diet. We don't have to give up our favorite foods to achieve a "healthy" status. I will declare it here; I am never giving up French fries! And you shouldn't give up the foods you love. Instead, choose balance over restriction. Choose healthy foods more than "unhealthy" options. Choose a dietary pattern that is easy to follow.

I want to share with you the dietary advice I give my clients. Below is a sample dietary pattern that is easy to follow and has been an effective meal plan for weight loss and maintaining a healthy body weight.

Breakfast: Whole grains and fruit

Lunch: 3-6 ounces of lean protein and 2 cups of vegetables

Dinner: 4-8 ounces of lean protein and 2 cups of vegetables

Snacks: fruit, nuts, protein (such as hard-boiled eggs or leftover chicken from lunch)

That's it, folks! Yes, it is a simple meal plan, but very effective. Breakfast means to "break fast." You are fasting while you sleep, and starting your day with foods that provide nutrients, fiber, and energy is essential. I prefer sprouted whole grains, which retain more nutrients and fiber. I will explain more about sprouted grains on Day 3. Fruit is also an excellent source of fiber, nutrients, and antioxidants. Here are examples for breakfast:

- Oatmeal, walnuts, and fruit

grain English muffin with peanut butter and uree

with rolled oats, cashews, and mixed berries

inner simple with your favorite protein, such ork, or grass-fed beef. Choose from a variety of vegetables to accompany your protein. Here are examples of lunch and dinner:

Lunch:

- 3-6 ounces of grilled chicken and two cups of mixed greens, or
- Omelet with spinach, mushroom, and tomatoes, or
- Bowl of vegetable soup and one slice of pita bread with hummus

Dinner:

- Grilled salmon, baked sweet potato, and string beans, or
- Skirt steak with grilled asparagus and roasted carrots, or
- Baked chicken with a side salad and garlic-roasted broccoli

Following my straightforward plan of grains and fruit for breakfast and lean protein and veggies for lunch and dinner will provide a balanced diet, including a variety of vitamins and minerals, fiber, lean protein, and healthy fat. The best part is that you get to choose the protein, fruits, and veggies. Choose *your favorite* fruit, grain, veggies, and lean protein in this simple diet pattern.

You may notice that some of your favorite food items are missing from this plan. For example, white bread, cereals, chips, and ice cream. These foods are usually the culprit of weight gain, so let's set these aside for the time being, and I will revisit how you can incorporate these foods on another day.

It is important to understand that you can train your body to react a certain way. For example, if you restrict calories and nutrients, your body will respond by slowing down due to a lack of energy and motivation. On the other hand, your body will thrive if you provide consistent sources of healthy nutrients and calories. Depriving your body of nutrients and calories by following a fad diet will not create healthy habits that lead to your overall health goal. But, consuming a diet that is loaded with nutrients and does not deprive your body of calories will help you to lose weight. It sounds weird that eating more will cause you to lose weight, but it is true – as long as you eat more of the good stuff and have the not-so-good stuff in moderation.

The meal pattern I shared will give you more energy. You will feel more creative and productive and feel good about yourself. When you feel good about yourself, you will continue to make healthy choices. You are on your way to achieving limitless health.

Today, I encourage you to try a new eating pattern. I understand that changing your entire diet at one time can be challenging, so start with one meal. If you feel ambitious, make 2-3 changes or change it all at once! The choice is yours.

Summary:

- A fad diet is a popular dietary pattern known as a quick fix for weight loss.

- Fad diets promise immediate results that require little effort but are often unattainable and unrealistic long-term.

- Restricting calories is effective for short-term weight loss. However, omitting a food group will result in more than fewer calories; your diet will be less nutritious, leading to nutrient deficiencies.

- Ditch diets and instead follow a straightforward plan of grains and fruit for breakfast and lean protein and veggies for lunch and dinner to receive a variety of vitamins and minerals, fiber, and healthy fat daily.

Achievable Actions:

Try at least one new meal pattern today:

- Breakfast: includes whole grains and fruit
- Lunch: 3-6 ounces of lean protein and 2 cups of vegetables
- Dinner: 4-8 ounces of lean protein and 2 cups of vegetables
- Snacks: fruit, nuts, protein (such as hard-boiled eggs or leftover chicken)

Day 3

I Love Carbs

Yesterday I asked you to ditch the diet mindset, which may include thinking potatoes are bad for you and baby carrots are loaded with sugar. Today, I am introducing you to the three macronutrients, but I will primarily focus on carbohydrates and why it is okay to love carbs. People continue to debate whether carbs are good or bad for you. Claims have been made that carbs will cause weight gain and diabetes and are downright evil. So, I am giving you the scoop about carbs and why you should include them in your diet every day.

Macronutrients, or "macros," are nutrients your body needs, including carbohydrates (carbs), protein, and fat. The macros provide your body with energy, in the form of calories, to function throughout the day. We need energy to move, digest a meal, regulate body temperature, and even dream. We obtain calories from food, and the body converts calories into usable energy via a process called cellular respiration. Within each of our cells is the ability to convert calories to energy. The amount of energy from calories a body needs varies depending on the individual. Factors such as age, gender, body weight, height, and physical activity affect how many calories we should consume daily from food. The calories of each macronutrient are as follows:

- Carbohydrates: 4 calories per gram
- Protein: 4 calories per gram
- Fat: 9 calories per gram

For example, if you consume a food source that includes 20 grams of protein, you will receive 80 calories from protein for that food. Men need about 2500 calories daily, and women need approximately 1800 calories daily to maintain weight. However, the number of calories can be adjusted for individuals who want to gain or lose weight. *Please visit www.tammyfogarty.com for more information about calories, how much you need, and how to decipher the food label.*

During digestion, carbohydrates are broken down into glucose, a simple carb. Think of glucose as fuel for your body, just as gasoline is fuel for your car. Glucose is a vital energy source, and your body prefers to use glucose for energy; in fact, the brain relies heavily on energy produced from glucose.

The amount of glucose in your body is detected from a blood test and is referred to as blood glucose or, as my family likes to call it, "sugar." After digestion, the body will utilize glucose for energy, and the remaining is stored in the liver and muscles as glycogen for later use. In addition, the body can quickly use glycogen for energy, allowing the body to always have fuel on hand. This comes in handy when we need to move or react quickly.

If I were to ask you to list foods that contain carbohydrates, what would you include? Pizza, pasta, rice, and bread are common responses when I ask this question. And yes, these are carbohydrates, but so are fruits, vegetables, legumes, dairy, and beans. There are two different categories of carbs: simple and complex.

Simple carbs are sugars. While some of these occur naturally in milk and fruit, most simple carbs are added to foods. They include:

- White sugar
- Brown sugar
- High-fructose corn syrup
- Fruit juice concentrate
- Glucose, fructose, and sucrose

Simple carbohydrate food sources to limit include:

- Baked goods (cookies, cakes, pastries)
- Juice from concentrate
- Soda
- Breakfast cereals

Complex carbs are more nutritious and contain fiber and starches. Fiber-rich, complex carbs include:

- Fruit
- Vegetables
- Whole Grains
- Beans

Complex carbs that contain less fiber are starchy grains and vegetables such as:

- Whole wheat bread
- Potatoes
- Oats
- Rice
- Corn
- Peas

Complex carbs to eat daily:

- Whole grains
- Fruit

- Vegetables
- Beans
- Legumes

The list above includes just a few examples of simple vs. complex carbohydrates, but you get the picture. Please visit www.tammyfogarty.com for a list of online nutrition courses.

Yesterday, I encouraged you to consume whole grains for breakfast. A grain in its natural state is referred to as a whole grain. A whole grain kernel includes the bran, germ, and endosperm. The bran (outer layer) and germ (inner layer) are concentrated sources of fiber, minerals, vitamins, and antioxidants. The endosperm is the center layer of the grain and is rich in starch and protein. The bran and germ are removed during refining, the process in which the endosperm is used to create refined flour, such as all-purpose flour. Here is the clincher: removing the bran and germ removes the healthiest part of the grain, leaving you with a calorie-dense food source used to make most of the processed, starchy foods that line the grocery store's shelves, such as bread, cereal, and pasta.

The most nutritious carbohydrates include fruit, vegetables, whole grains, and beans. Whole grains include barley, oats, millet, quinoa, and brown rice. Enjoy a variety of fruits and vegetables, and add beans to soups and salads.

The carbs you want to limit are those made from refined flour and sugar, such as cakes, pastries, cookies, white bread, and most cereals. Of course, it is even better to omit them altogether, but enjoying these foods occasionally is perfectly acceptable.

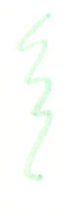

As I mentioned on Day 2, focusing on overall food quality is important. Having a slice of white toast for breakfast is not the issue, but having a diet that consists of mostly refined, processed foods is of concern because you are receiving calories without any nutrients. In addition, refined grains are quickly digested, converted to glucose, and used as energy. As a result, blood glucose levels rapidly spike, followed by a dramatic drop, leaving you hungry shortly after a meal.

On the flip side, a meal consisting of whole grains, including fiber, protein, vitamins, and minerals, is digested at a slower rate, providing a steady release of glucose into the blood and releasing energy consistently. Whole grains and vegetables do not cause spikes in blood glucose levels due to their fiber content and will not leave you tired and ready for an afternoon nap. Whole grains provide long-lasting energy that will make you feel full after a meal.

Lastly, a balanced diet that includes whole grains reduces the risk of diabetes, cardiovascular disease, and high blood pressure and helps maintain a healthy weight. In contrast, a diet high in refined grains is associated with weight gain, increasing the risk of diabetes, obesity, elevated triglycerides contributing to heart disease, and inflammation that can trigger inflammatory bowel conditions and arthritis. Therefore, the issue of whether or not to eat or ditch carbohydrates from the diet is complex. We tend to lump foods into a one-size-fits-all category; clearly, not all carbs are the same, and we are all unique individuals with varying needs. It is essential to find what works for your body and stop listening to the noise and fad diets telling you how and what to eat.

If you still have reservations about having a loving relationship with carbs, how about we dive into some of the most common carb myths?

Carb Myth #1: Carbs make you fat — FALSE

The most popular sources of carbohydrates are starchy carbs. Bread, pasta, and rice are examples of starchy carbs, and unfortunately, starchy carbs are higher in calories per serving. For example, a cup of pasta provides approximately 200 calories, but who eats just one cup of pasta? A typical plate of pasta includes 2-4 cups, so you can see how easily the calories add up. However, leafy greens (don't forget that veggies are carbs) provide only 25-65 calories per cup; 1-2 cups is a typical serving for a side salad of leafy greens. So, our pasta meal can add up to 800 calories compared to 50 calories of leafy salad greens.

Just because the most loved carbohydrates tend to contain more calories does not mean that they are solely responsible for weight gain or that you have to give them up. Instead, eat a dinner serving of salad (3-4 cups) and a smaller portion of pasta (1-2 cups). Remember, the salad provides fiber and nutrients that will leave you feeling full and curb your desire to indulge in a big bowl of pasta.

Carb Myth #2: All carbs turn to sugar — TRUE

Regardless of the food source, carbohydrates will break down into glucose, a simple sugar, during digestion. But not all carbs are created equal, and you cannot compare a candy bar to a piece of fruit. For example, my favorite candy bar is Snickers, which contains several refined ingredients, including sugar and chocolate, whereas one of my favorite fruits, strawberries, contains fiber, vitamins, and antioxidants. Therefore, there is no comparison, and the sugar you get from strawberries, known as fructose, is not associated with an increased risk of disease. In contrast, the Snickers bar contains ingredients that, when consumed in excess, have been associated with conditions such as heart disease, obesity, and diabetes. When was the last time you heard of someone gaining weight because they ate too many strawberries?

Again, it is important to focus on the overall quality of the diet. I shake my head when anyone tells me they can't eat fruit because it contains too much sugar. And I can't blame them; they probably heard this fruit-hating myth from someone who preferred to eat candy bars rather than snack on grapes. So, eat the fruit and the baby carrots with reckless abandon. And enjoy the candy bar every once in a while.

Carb Myth #3: Eating too much sugar causes diabetes — FALSE

Eating sugar does not cause diabetes. That's right, folks. You heard it here. True story. Let's refer back to diet quality. Consuming foods regularly that contain refined grains and sugar contributes to weight gain, thus promoting insulin resistance, which may result in the development of type 2 diabetes. The American Heart Association recommends no more than 38 grams (9 teaspoons) of added sugar for men and 25 grams (6 teaspoons) of added sugar for women daily. Added sugar refers to refined sugar or syrups added to foods during preparation, processing, or at the table. Naturally occurring sugars are found *naturally* in foods such as fruit (fructose and glucose) and milk (lactose). For example, plain yogurt will contain about 8 grams of sugar from lactose, a sugar found naturally in milk. In comparison, fruit-flavored yogurt contains jam and can have up to 18-25 grams of added sugar.

If you are concerned about developing diabetes, limit processed foods containing refined grains and sugar and get your heart pumping. A sedentary lifestyle has been associated with an increased risk of type 2 diabetes. So, grab an apple and take a walk, nothing crazy, but a better option than a cupcake on the couch.

Carb Myth #4: You will lose weight if you cut carbs — TRUE

Sure, water weight. A function of carbs is in its name, carbo-HYDRATE. The origin of the term "carbohydrate" is based on its components: carbon ("carbo") and water ("hydrate"). The mechanism that causes the body to lose weight is two-fold:

glycogen and insulin. As carbohydrate intake decreases, so do glycogen and insulin, so let's make sense of it all.

The body stores carbs as glycogen, which binds to water in the muscles and liver. When carbohydrate intake decreases, the body will use stored glycogen for energy by converting it back to glucose. This process releases water; therefore, the initial weight loss seen in the first two weeks is water loss. However, when you consume carbs again, your body will retain water.

In addition, a low-carb diet is associated with less sodium intake due to the omission of refined grains and snack foods. The result of decreased carb intake is a reduction of insulin. Insulin is a hormone that transports glucose into the cells to produce energy, but insulin also retains sodium. When you retain sodium, you're going to retain water. As a result, when insulin levels decrease, the kidneys remove excess sodium from the body. This also helps to lower blood pressure. In a nutshell, processed foods contain sodium. When you decrease the amount of processed foods from your diet, you will retain less sodium, thus you will lose water weight and also lower your blood pressure. It's a win-win situation!

Let's revisit diet quality one more time. Refined, starchy carbohydrates such as bread, pasta, cereals, and baked goods are calorically dense foods with minimal nutrition. Limiting these foods is not only a nutritionally wise decision but may also promote weight loss. A diet that includes fruit, vegetables, whole grains, and beans is an excellent source of carbohydrates, providing the body with energy, nutrients, and antioxidants.

The type of carbohydrates you choose to eat daily will dictate your well-being. I suggest eating foods in their natural state (fruits, veggies, whole grains) and limiting the number of processed foods. If your food can live on a shelf in a grocery store for an extended period of time, it is safe to say that you should consume it in moderation. Or better yet, just avoid it.

The foods you should consume are those that can rot. Yes, you read that right. Fruit, veggies, meat, poultry, fish, and dairy will eventually rot because they are *natural*. Rotting is a natural process. If your food does not rot and can live in your pantry for a year, you may want to think twice about eating it. Mother Nature has lovingly provided us with all we need: foods that do not require preservatives or a food scientist to mastermind a chemically crafted, artificially flavored food. So, go on. Love your carbs. The right carbs.

Here is the ideal meal pattern that I shared on Day 2 so that you can see how easy it is to incorporate a variety of nutrient-dense carbohydrates into our meals:

Breakfast:

- Oatmeal, walnuts, and fruit
- Sprouted whole grain English muffin with peanut butter and sliced strawberries
- Smoothie with rolled oats, cashews, and mixed berries

Lunch:

- 3-6 ounces of grilled chicken and two cups of mixed greens
- Omelet with spinach, mushroom, and tomatoes
- Bowl of vegetable soup and one slice of pita bread and hummus

Dinner:

- Grilled salmon, baked sweet potato, and string beans
- Skirt steak with grilled asparagus and roasted carrots
- Baked chicken with a side salad and garlic-roasted broccoli

Approximately 45-65% of your daily calories should come from carbohydrates. The amount depends on how physically active you are. So, if you do not exercise, you can stick to about 45% of

==your calories from carbs and increase it to about 50-55% of your calories as you become more physically active.==

I want to leave you with one last piece of advice when choosing foods. Balance. Balance is key. My metabolism was at its all-time best when I was in high school. I didn't think twice about eating 3 or 4 slices of pizza. I loved it, and I ate a lot of pizza. However, while earning my nutrition degree, I followed a strict vegetarian lifestyle and wouldn't dream of eating pizza. After all, I was going to be a nutritionist, and in my mind, the best way to lead by example was to avoid all refined foods and shame others when they made "unhealthy" choices. I admit, this was not my finest moment, but with experience came the knowledge I carry today.

Today, balance means enjoying a slice or two of pizza because I still *love* pizza. But instead of filling up solely on pizza, I have a salad, too. I enjoy the salad as much as the pizza because it is the food that nourishes my mind and body. It makes me feel good, and I enjoy the pizza much more. So, find your balance. Enjoy the foods you love, but find the right balance so your body can benefit from your choices.

Carbohydrates are not evil. They are a necessity as they provide the fuel the body requires to function. Place fruit, vegetables, and whole grains on your list of go-to carbs to fuel your body. Enjoy refined carbohydrates in moderation. Moderation to me means 1-2 times per week, sometimes less, and certainly, there are times when I consume more. Again, it's about balance and finding what works for you.

If you have a limited palette and hate eating fruits and vegetables, or can't even fathom the thought of eating legumes or beans; I encourage you to *try*. You are reading this book because you want to live a healthy life. I bet you don't hate all vegetables and beans. Instead, you may hate the way your mom prepared them when you were a child. I get it! I gagged on mashed potatoes and had a meltdown at the mere sight of anything green, but I love these foods today. The mashed potatoes my grandmother made felt like a ball of goop in my mouth, and vegetables were cooked until they were a wilted heap of food that resembled parrot shit on my plate.

I am sure you can relate, but it's time to put on your big kid pants and expand your food horizon. I hated the texture and consistency of certain foods and didn't enjoy vegetables until I was in my twenties and learned to prepare them in a way that enhanced the flavor. Roasted veggies are among my favorite things to eat now, and I eat veggies with just about every meal. And, bring on the mashed potatoes!! Mine are light and fluffy. I can go as far as saying they are a healthy comfort food for me.

So, if you don't like something, try eating it a new way. Do yourself a favor and don't just turn your nose up to food, especially an entire food group. Try new recipes, experiment with different cooking methods such as grilling and roasting, and have fun with flavors. The addition of fresh herbs to any dish will make your taste buds dance a happy dance. And who doesn't love a happy dance?

Summary:

- Macronutrients, or "macros," are nutrients your body needs, including carbohydrates (carbs), protein, and fat.
- The macros provide your body with energy so that you can function throughout the day.
- Simple carbs are sugars. While some occur naturally in milk and fruit, most simple carbs are added to foods such as white sugar and high fructose corn syrup.

- Complex carbs are more nutritious and contain fiber and starches. Fiber-rich, complex carbs include fruit, vegetables, whole grains, and beans.

- Complex carbs that contain less fiber are starchy grains and vegetables such as whole wheat bread, potatoes, and oats.

- Refined, starchy carbohydrates such as bread, pasta, cereals, and baked goods are calorically dense foods with minimal nutrition. Limiting these foods is not only a nutritionally wise decision but may also promote weight loss.

- A diet that includes fruit, vegetables, whole grains, and beans is an excellent source of carbohydrates, providing the body with energy, nutrients, and antioxidants. The type of carbohydrates you choose to eat daily will dictate your well-being.

Achievable Actions:

- Choose 2-3 complex carbohydrates that you will add to your meal plan today.

- Choose to eliminate 1-2 refined, processed carbohydrates from your day.

- Try a new way to prepare food that you don't typically care for.

Day 4

The Skinny on Fats

Today, I want you to love fats as much as you love carbs right now. And, just as with carbohydrates, not all fats are created equal. By the end of this day, you will differentiate between the good fats, the bad fats, and everything in between. Knowing the difference can help you determine which fats you should include and which you should limit in your diet.

Fun Fat Facts:

- Fats are found in plant and animal foods.
- Certain fats are linked to cardiovascular disease, while others protect us from heart disease.
- Fats provide energy, nine calories per gram.
- Fats are required to absorb fat-soluble vitamins A, D, E, and K.
- Fat in the body protects and cushions your vital organs.
- Fat regulates body temperature.
- Healthy fats are anti-inflammatory.
- Fats can optimize brain function.
- A meal that includes healthy fats will help prevent spikes in blood sugar.
- Fats may improve your skin health.

Fats are characterized by their molecular structure as saturated or unsaturated fat. Saturated fats are often considered "unhealthy" and can cause health concerns when consumed in excess. Unsaturated fats promote heart health and thus are considered "healthy" fat sources. It is important to note that all foods containing fat have a mixture of saturated and unsaturated fats. Not one food contains a single source of dietary fat; therefore, enjoy a variety of foods to ensure you receive the benefits of fat.

Saturated Fat

Most saturated fat comes from animal-based foods. Saturated fat is also found in plant-based foods like coconut and palm oil. Foods that contain saturated fat include:

- Fatty cuts of beef, pork, lamb, bacon
- Dark meat poultry, poultry skin
- High-fat dairy foods such as cheese, ice cream, sour cream, whole milk
- Butter, lard, coconut oil, palm oil, palm kernel oil
- Baked goods containing refined sugar, refined wheat, excess fat, and trans fat

Excess saturated fat intake is associated with a risk of heart disease and certain cancers; however, research is continually evolving, and what we know today is much different than the advice followed thirty years ago. The American Heart Association recommends that no more than 5% to 6% of calories should come from saturated fat. For example, if you follow a 2,000-calorie diet, no more than 120 calories, or approximately 13 grams, should come from saturated fat. Don't be afraid to enjoy foods containing saturated fats, just don't go overboard.

Unsaturated Fat

Unsaturated fats can improve blood cholesterol levels, reduce inflammation, and protect from heart disease. Unsaturated fats are predominantly found in plant foods, such as plant-based oils, nuts, and seeds. There are two types of unsaturated fats: monounsaturated and polyunsaturated.

Examples of monounsaturated fats are:

- Avocados
- Nuts such as almonds, cashews, peanuts, and pecans
- Seeds such as pumpkin, sesame, and sunflower seeds
- Olive, peanut, and avocado oil

Examples of polyunsaturated fats are:

- Sunflower and flaxseed oil
- Walnuts
- Flaxseed
- Fish

Omega-3 and omega-6 fatty acids are essential fatty acids because your body needs them to function properly but is unable to produce them on its own. That means you must obtain them from your diet. Omega-3 fatty acids include fish, walnuts, flax seeds, flaxseed oil, and chia seeds. They help regulate blood pressure, and irregular heart rate, and reduce inflammation.

Omega-6 fatty acids are found in safflower oil, mayonnaise, nuts, seeds, poultry, fish, meat, and eggs. Omega-6 fatty acids maintain the structure and function of your cells and lower LDL while boosting the production of HDL.

Trans Fat

Trans fatty acids, or trans fats, are formed when food manufacturers turn liquid oils into solid fats. Think of turning vegetable oil into margarine. Trans fats are created via hydrogenation, a process by which vegetable oils are converted to solid fats by adding hydrogen atoms. Trans fats were developed during the backlash when animal fats, found in butter, cream, and meats, were considered "bad for you." As a result, today, trans fats are found in 40% of the products on your supermarket shelves. Unfortunately, trans fat has negative effects on the body. It is the worst type of fat for heart disease and is associated with inflammation, elevated LDL cholesterol, and insulin resistance; therefore, it is recommended to avoid foods that contain trans fats. Trans fats are commonly found in:

- Packaged baked goods made with hydrogenated oils such as cookies, cupcakes, and granola bars
- Processed snack foods such as crackers and microwave popcorn
- Margarine
- Shortening
- Fried foods such as French fries and doughnuts
- Non-dairy creamer
- Frozen pizza
- Refrigerated dough such as biscuits and pie crust

The good news is that trans fats are easily identified by reading the food label. Food labels must list the amount of trans fat in food, and you can identify trans fats by looking for "hydrogenated" or "partially hydrogenated" oils in the list of ingredients.

The main health concern with dietary fat, which has been widely researched, is how it may influence cholesterol levels. Consuming high amounts of saturated fat produces more LDL (bad) cholesterol, resulting in plaque formation in the arteries, thus increasing the risk of cardiovascular disease and stroke. In comparison, unsaturated fats help increase HDL (good) cholesterol levels, removing excess LDL in the blood by transporting it to the liver for later use (or for discard).

Despite decades of dietary advice that saturated fats are harmful, current research suggests that eating diets high in saturated fat does not raise the risk of heart disease. So, we face a crossroads of how much fat is too much. We know that a diet containing healthy fats, in place of saturated fat, lowers the "bad" LDL cholesterol, raises the "good" HDL cholesterol, and improves the ratio of total cholesterol, thus lowering the risk of heart disease.

The benefits of heart-healthy fats include:

- Decreasing the risk of developing heart disease
- Improving blood cholesterol levels
- Stabilizing blood sugar by slowing the absorption of blood glucose after a meal
- Promoting satiety, which makes you feel full and satisfied after a meal
- Reducing inflammation
- Supporting gut health
- Enhancing the immune system

Unfortunately, many of us don't get adequate amounts of healthy fats. But today, you can turn that around by including sources of unsaturated fat, limiting excess saturated fats, avoiding trans fats, and eating at least one good source of omega-3 fats each day.

Today, you will enjoy healthy sources of fat along with your complex carbohydrates. The combination of fat and complex carbohydrates prevents spikes in blood sugar. And this is great because spikes in blood sugar are responsible for that sluggish feeling you get after a meal. Fat and carbs together will leave you feeling energized and satisfied after a meal and make you feel fuller for longer periods. This is a good thing, especially if weight loss is your goal. What fats will you choose to add to your diet today?

Summary:

- Fats are characterized by their molecular structure as saturated or unsaturated fat.

- Saturated fats are often considered "unhealthy" and can cause health concerns when consumed in excess.

- Unsaturated fats promote heart health and are "healthy" fat sources.

- Despite decades of dietary advice that saturated fats are harmful, current research suggests that eating diets high in saturated fat does not raise the risk of heart disease.

- A diet containing healthy fats, in place of saturated fat, lowers the "bad" LDL cholesterol, raises the "good" HDL cholesterol, and improves the ratio of total cholesterol, thus lowering the risk of heart disease.

Achievable Actions:

- Choose 1-2 healthy fats to incorporate into your diet.

- Choose at least one food source that contains excess saturated fat that you can limit in your diet, such as margarine, cookies, pastries, and cheese.

- Avoid foods that contain trans fats.

Day 5

Protein: It's So Much More Than Building Muscles

Most people associate protein with building big, strong muscles. There is some truth in that statement; however, protein plays a much bigger role than you may think and is involved in almost every metabolic function of your body. Protein surely doesn't get the credit it deserves, yet people feel the need to eat it like it's going out of style. Everyone is going crazy eating protein and taking supplements! Today, you will learn the top five things you should know about protein and why you don't need to jump on the protein bandwagon. You will also better understand why we don't need to eat a side of beef to build biceps.

Protein is an essential macronutrient, and, much like fat and carbs, not all protein is created equal. *Do you notice a trend here?* Protein is made of twenty amino acids, known as the body's building blocks because protein helps to build the body. Protein is responsible for building bones, tissues, organs, enzymes... you name it, and protein plays a role in it. Nine of the twenty amino acids are essential and must come from food. The remaining are produced in the body, known as the non-essential amino acids.

The Recommended Dietary Allowance for healthy adults is 0.8 grams per kilogram of body weight or roughly 7 grams per 20 pounds. For example, a person weighing 140 pounds needs approximately 50 grams of protein daily. Protein requirements are relatively high during periods of growth, such as childhood and pregnancy, but outside of growing and pregnancy, it's important to have consistent intake in the right amounts. Protein requirements are higher for athletes, but I will elaborate on this subject in a moment.

We obtain protein from two sources: animal and plant-based sources of food. Animal-based sources of protein include:

- Beef
- Poultry
- Fish
- Eggs
- Pork

Examples of plant-based proteins include:

- Nuts
- Beans
- Seeds
- Tofu
- Legumes
- Grains

The function of protein includes:

- Production of muscle and structural tissues
- Required for bone growth
- Transports molecules
- Required for the production of enzymes and hormones

- Used to make antibodies to protect the body
- Make up the structural components of cells and tissue
- Needed for the growth of hair, nails, and skin
- Maintains fluid balance and pH

Body proteins are continually being repaired and replaced. This process, known as protein synthesis, requires a continuous supply of amino acids. This means we must eat dietary protein to meet our body's amino acid demand.

Protein and Exercise

Protein is necessary for building and repairing muscles. However, consuming more protein than the body can utilize will not give you bigger, better, and stronger muscles. In fact, too much protein will be converted and stored as fat. While research shows that protein consumption after a workout aids muscle repair and growth, most individuals consume more protein than the body can use.

Tiny tears in the muscle fibers result when you do weight-bearing activities, such as lifting weights. The role of protein is to repair the muscle for continued use. The body's ability to recover after a workout requires adequate rest and proper nutrition. An important component of the recovery process is consuming both carbohydrates and protein shortly after exercise to restore muscle glycogen (stored carbs we discussed on Day 3) and stimulate muscle protein synthesis. Fueling your workout with food that adequately supports your favorite activities is essential. To ensure you are ready for physical activity, use the EAT guidelines:

Eat breakfast. The best way to start the day is by eating breakfast. Include foods that contain carbohydrates and protein, such as whole grains, yogurt, and eggs.

Add carbohydrates and protein after a workout. Carbohydrates replenish muscle glycogen stores, and protein helps build and repair muscles.

Toss the supplements. The goal is to obtain protein from food sources instead of relying on supplements or protein shakes. Doing so will ensure a balanced diet and better prepare you for physical performance.

Remember, eating more protein does not create stronger, bigger muscles. You do this by engaging in regular physical activities. To increase your muscle mass, you must engage in weight-bearing activity. You can bulk up muscle mass by increasing the weight and repetitions over time. So, keep up the good work. And make sure to include good protein sources in your diet to repair and replete your muscles.

Protein Supplements

Protein supplements are marketed to help promote muscle growth, enhance physical performance, boost energy, and support weight loss. Supplements are available as powders, bars, and shakes and are a convenient way to get more protein. But are they necessary? Since most people already eat plenty of protein, adding a protein supplement is unnecessary.

Adding extra protein to a meal or snack is the best way to boost your intake if you need more protein. Excellent sources of protein include fish, eggs, poultry, meat, tofu, beans, and nuts. And protein-rich foods naturally contain the fiber, vitamins, and minerals to keep healthy. You won't get that from a protein supplement.

If you decide to take protein supplements, remember that they may contain added sugars and fat that will increase your caloric intake, leading to weight gain. Supplements are meant to 'supplement' a balanced diet, not replace it. Foods first, but if you must take supplements, read the label so you know what you are taking.

Top 5 things you should know about protein:

1. **Protein is not just for muscle growth.** Protein is required to produce hormones, enzymes, maintain proper pH, balance fluid in the body, and is a vital component of every cell in your body.

2. **Plant-based proteins are a good source of protein.** Proteins from plant-based sources are considered "incomplete" proteins because they do not contain all essential amino acids, as with animal-based proteins. However, consuming a balanced diet of beans, nuts, seeds, and grains will provide the essential amino acids that can be used to create non-essential amino acids. These amino acids, in turn, will link together in a specific sequence to produce a body protein needed to make our cells, tissues, skin, hair, nails, enzymes, etc. The key to a healthy plant-based diet is to include a variety of foods to achieve a balanced diet.

3. **Protein gives your immune system a boost.** Adequate protein intake is necessary to give your body the tools to fight viruses and bacterial infections. The antibodies that fight infection and foreign invaders are made up of protein. In addition, foods that are a good source of protein often contain other micronutrients that boost immunity, such as magnesium in almonds and zinc in red meat.

4. **Protein supplements should not replace food sources of protein.** Protein supplements should be used to 'supplement' your diet when you cannot obtain sufficient protein from food. However, food sources of protein should always be your first choice as it provides you with

a variety of vitamins, minerals, and antioxidants not found in commercial powders, bars, and supplements.

5. **A high-protein diet is not all it's cracked up to be.** The key to a healthy diet is balance. Avoid focusing on one macronutrient. Fats, protein, and carbs all provide essential nutrients, and each macro plays a significant role in the body. Eat various foods that contain healthy fats, complex carbs, and protein to achieve optimal nutrition. Remember that too much of anything is not a good thing. And excess protein, beyond what your body needs, is converted and stored as fat.

What's on your agenda today? Hopefully, you will enhance your plate by adding lean protein from animal and plant-based sources. As I mentioned yesterday, each meal should include a complex carbohydrate and healthy fat. Today, you will add protein to each meal, too. Like with fat, protein also maintains normal blood sugar levels by preventing spikes in sugar. I advise including complex carbs, healthy fat, and protein at each meal. Bon appetit!

Summary:

- Protein is an essential macronutrient.

- Protein is responsible for building bones, tissues, organs, enzymes... you name it, and protein plays a role in it.

- The Recommended Dietary Allowance for healthy adults is 0.8 grams per kilogram of body weight or roughly 7 grams per 20 pounds.

- Protein is necessary for rebuilding and repairing muscles. However, consuming more protein than the body can utilize will not give you bigger and stronger muscles.

- It is essential to fuel your workout with food that adequately supports your favorite activities.

Achievable Actions:

- Include 2-3 plant-based protein sources in your diet.

- Choose a pre- and post-workout snack that contains carbohydrates and protein to fuel your activity.

- Create a healthy meal by choosing a complex carbohydrate, lean protein, and healthy fat.

Day 6

Shhhh... Your Body Is Trying to Tell You Something

You may have already tried a diet or, in most cases, have tried a variety of different types of diets. You may be following influencers on social media. Most likely, you have purchased a workout plan, meal plan, or any plan that promises to help you reach your ultimate goal. But remember that fad diets, meal plans, and workout plans *tell* you what to do rather than explain how and why you should eat a certain way or do a specific exercise. This is one of the reasons why diets don't work. And, let's face it, most adults do not want to be told what to do and eventually return to their old routines.

Remember that routines are comfortable and familiar. But you are reading this book because you are looking for guidance and are ready to create a new healthy routine. But to do so, you need to make a big leap and be able to sit with feeling uncomfortable. You must also be brutally honest with yourself. When you make time to be honest with yourself, sit with discomfort, and take action to change, you will open the doors to healing and living your limitless potential. And don't worry, you won't feel uncomfortable for long. You will feel the best you have felt in a long time.

Are you ready to welcome change? Are you ready to learn what to eat to feel better? Okay, you got it! But you must listen closely because it is not coming from me. It is coming from *your body*.

Did you know that your brain and gut talk to each other? It's called the Brain-Gut Axis. Your brain and gut can communicate via hormones, known as chemical messengers. For example, we receive messages daily when we are hungry or full. We also get those "gut feelings" or intuition when we feel strongly about a situation. This communication, or cross-talk, between the brain and the gut sends cues throughout the day, such as when to eat and when to stop. We also receive cues responsible for food cravings, and the brain-gut axis sends signals that can affect our mood. I will dive deeper into the brain-gut axis later in this book. Today, I want you to get friendly with your body and learn how to identify the cues your body so lovingly sends all day.

Let's start by taking a moment to think about your last meal. Take a mental note of where you were and what you did during your meal. Did you notice how you felt before and after your meal?

If you are scratching your head, saying, "I don't know," then you are not alone. Most of us do not take the time to assess our surroundings and feelings before and after we eat. Usually, we dig in without thinking about it, until today. Today, you will practice my favorite and the most effective tool I share with my clients: Mindful Eating. This strategy allows you to "listen" to the communication between your brain and your gut. Once you have mastered this, you will determine how foods make you feel and how to avoid overeating.

Mindful Eating allows you to assess how you feel before and during your meal and how food makes you feel afterward. But to do this exercise, you must follow a few simple rules when you sit down for your next meal.

- Step 1: **Assess how you feel**. Assess if you feel hungry. Often, we eat because it is a specific time of day or because food is present. So, take a moment to assess your hunger level and why you are preparing to eat. If you are not feeling hungry, pour yourself a glass of water and wait until your body signals the need for energy (aka food). If you are hungry, proceed to step 2.

- Step 2: **Shut it down**. Electronics distract us, so it is vital to disconnect from any distractions. Put your phone away, turn off the television, and look away from your computer. Don't worry; you will be okay without your phone for a few minutes. The goal is to shut everything down so that you are completely mindful and present as you begin your meal.

- Step 3: **Prepare your plate**. For this exercise, you will section your plate into three portions. You don't have to divide your food; however, please take a mental note of your plate because you will eat ⅓ of your plate at a time. And, if you are like me and hate math, ⅓ + ⅓ + ⅓ = 100%. So, let's get started with the first portion of your meal in step 4.

- Step 4: **Eat slowly**. This step will take a little time, but it is worth it. Take your first bite, put your fork down, and chew your food slowly. We tend to add more food into our mouths before swallowing what is there. Therefore, placing your fork down is a crucial step to avoid mindless shoveling of food into your mouth. Savor each bite, taste your food, and take your time. Scientists say we should chew each bite 32 times. A bonus of chewing your food well is that it improves digestion. Enjoy your meal, one sweet bite at a time.

- Step 5: **Gauge your hunger level.** After you eat the first portion of your meal, sit back and take about three minutes to assess your hunger level. This is when your brain and gut communicate. But, if we don't stop eating, we can't listen to what our body tells us. So, sit back, relax, and listen. Do you feel hungry, satisfied, or full? If you are hungry, continue to step 6. If you feel satisfied or full, put the remaining food in a container and enjoy it as a snack or meal later in the day.

- Step 6: **Eat slowly.** If you still feel hungry, eat the second portion of your meal. Again, be mindful of chewing each bite well and putting your fork down between bites.

- Step 7: **Gauge your hunger level.** Re-assess how you feel after eating two portions of your meal. After about three minutes, assess if you are hungry, satisfied, or full. If you are hungry, consume the last portion of your plate. But if you are feeling satisfied or full, stop eating. Remember, you don't have to eat until you are full. Feeling satisfied is just as good, if not better.

- Step 8: **Assess how you feel after a meal.** It's important to note how you feel after your meal. Are you feeling full or satisfied? Do you feel stuffed or comfortable? Be mindful of how you feel over the next few hours. Your energy level, productivity, and motivation are some things to consider.

This exercise aims to identify the cues your body sends you so that you eat when you are hungry rather than because of the time of day, the smell of something good, or boredom. As I mentioned earlier, our bodies prefer a routine, such as eating at specific times of the day. Routine is good, but it can cause you to eat when you are not hungry. For example, you may be required to take a lunch break at a specific time. But what if you are not hungry during your lunch break? I would advise eating something light to refuel your brain, such as fruit or vegetables with a heart-healthy dip like hummus or guacamole. Small snacks throughout the day are just as effective as consuming a meal. Most likely, you will have a break in the afternoon so you can use that time to refuel your engine (aka your brain). The most important thing is to be mindful of what your body needs: food, something to drink, or simply a mental break from the day.

What about if you just don't feel hungry? For example, some people don't feel hungry in the morning, so they choose not to eat. I challenge you to focus on why you are not receiving the cues to eat. For example, what is in your morning coffee? Depending on how much cream and sugar you use or how many cups you have, your morning cup of Joe can quickly add up to 300 calories and affect your appetite.

In addition, electronics, work, the kids, etc. are all distractions that will speak louder than our brain and gut can communicate. You may miss the communication your body sends if you are always busy and distracted. Take time for yourself and create an environment that fosters your ability to listen to your body's needs.

Mindful Eating aims to identify when you are hungry, had enough food, and how you feel. Your body is a well-oiled machine that sends messages telling you when to eat, what to eat via cravings, when to stop eating, and when to burn calories to maintain balance. Therefore, you do not need me to tell you what or how much to eat. Your brain and gut are in harmony and communicate effectively, informing you exactly what your body needs. Unfortunately, we live distracted lives and do not always listen. But when you begin listening, you will realize the profound connection between what you eat and how your body functions, especially the brain. Are you ready to start listening today?

You have at least three opportunities to eat intuitively throughout the day. Take time to enjoy your food and the opportunity to nourish your body. Taste each bite and its unique flavor. Feel the energy your foods provide. It's the perfect adult version of a time-out. As a result, your body will tell you exactly what it needs. If you listen closely, you will eat until you feel satisfied, creating an environment that promotes energy to foster creativity and productivity. *Please visit www.tammyfogarty.com to download your Mindful Eating journal.*

Summary:

- Diets, meal plans, and workout plans *tell* you what to do rather than teach you how to create a healthy eating behavior long-term.

- The brain and gut can communicate via our hormones.

- Get friendly with your body and learn how to identify the cues that your body so lovingly sends, all day, every day.

- Most of us do not take the time to assess our surroundings and feelings before and after we eat.

- Mindful Eating allows you to assess how you feel before and during your meal and how food makes you feel afterward.

Achievable Actions:

- Download the Mindful Eating Journal from www.tammyfogarty.com.

- Practice the Mindful Eating techniques at your next meal and note how you feel and, most importantly, how certain foods make you feel.

Day 7

Proactive, Not Reactive

As you know, I have a family history of breast cancer. A doctor once suggested I be proactive and have a mastectomy to remove my breasts, plus a hysterectomy. He told me that doing so would decrease my chances of developing cancer, like my mom. This news tugged at my heartstrings and made my head spin. And so I did what I do best: I researched.

In my research, I decided to speak with a geneticist to determine if I had a genetic predisposition to developing breast cancer. A genetic predisposition means an increased risk of a person developing a disease based on their genetic makeup. During my visit, she told me that 15% of diagnosed cases of diseases, such as heart disease, diabetes, and cancer, are related to genetics. The remaining 85% of cases are due to lifestyle choices.

Lifestyle choices! Let that sink in. It means you can do something daily that can impact the risk of developing a disease. **You have a choice in every moment.** Your choices include the foods you eat, how physically active you are, how you react to stress, the environment in which you live and work, and how much sleep you get each night. There are some factors that we cannot change, such as age, gender, and genetic makeup, but we can change our environment, which plays a significant role in genetic expression, or how these factors can turn genes on or off. Let's dive deeper into what we can control and how we can be more proactive.

The basic structure of our DNA is the building block for our genes, but not all genes behave the same. Your genes play an important role in your health, but so do your behaviors and environment, such as what you eat and how much you exercise. Epigenetics is the study of how your behaviors and environment can cause changes that affect the way your genes work or the processes that help direct when genes are turned on or off. For example, your dietary intake may turn off a specific gene related to cardiovascular disease, or a toxic environment may turn on a gene that leads to cancer development.

Additionally, researchers have found that early-life exposure to maternal dietary patterns, maternal stress, and environmental chemicals can increase the likelihood of developing disease later in life. Basically, the effects of poor diet, physical inactivity, stress, and the environment can be passed down from mom to baby and for multiple generations. So, your grandmother's lifestyle choices could affect how your genes behave today.

What would you do differently if you knew you had a genetic predisposition to a certain disease?

The response that I commonly hear is to eat healthy and exercise. Unfortunately, most people will wait until they are diagnosed with a disease to make a positive change. Why wait?

In 2009, my world got turned upside down. Allow me to provide a little insight. I met my first husband, Neil, when I was twenty and attending community college. Neil was eight years older than me and previously attended a University in Michigan where he played hockey and became involved in weightlifting. During this time, he experimented with steroids and consumed a high-protein diet designed for bodybuilders. His typical breakfast would be a dozen eggs with a pound of ground beef. Lunch and dinner would be about 12 ounces of chicken with a sweet potato and a head of broccoli. Dinner was typically a large steak with more broccoli. As a nutrition student, I questioned his eating habits, but he insisted this was how to build muscle. In his mind, nothing could go wrong.

Thankfully, he quit using steroids shortly after we began dating and reduced the daily amount of protein. However, his diet continued to be centered around animal protein. He rarely ate fruit or vegetables but did start eating more grains, usually cereal for breakfast and brown rice or couscous with dinner. We often prepared separate dinners since I focused on a plant-centered diet, and he was not ready to completely shift his routine. After all, he had consumed a high-protein diet for a while, and we all know that change can be challenging.

Over the years, Neil would complain of symptoms related to low blood sugar but refused to see a doctor despite my persistent requests that he get a physical. Eventually, he gave in and saw a doctor who was concerned with his blood sugar levels. He ordered a series of blood tests and an ultrasound to check his organs. Neil did not follow through and insisted he was fine. He did not want to be bothered with going to the lab or getting an ultrasound.

In the 13 years that we were together, Neil saw two doctors. I just mentioned one, and the second was a doctor specializing in men's health, specifically treating men who used steroids. Neil's hormone levels were low, and the doctor claimed that he could restore hormone balance and prescribed growth hormones to address abnormalities. I was concerned about the use of growth hormones and asked the doctor what would happen if, God forbid, there was a tumor. Because of my Mom, my mind always shifts to the "what if" scenario. I was concerned that hormones could accelerate tumor growth. The doctor assured us that cancer in a young man is highly unlikely and that if there were a rare chance of a tumor, the blood analysis would detect it. He said we had nothing to worry about.

About six months later, Neil feels good and has more energy, and we are planning our wedding after a seven-year engagement. I was ecstatic to get married. We planned a destination wedding in Napa Valley, California, and six weeks before our vows, I took a trip to California to meet with the vendors to finalize the wedding plans. The day after I left, Neil complained of stomach pains and took himself to the walk-in clinic. I knew it had to be serious for him to see a doctor. They diagnosed him with colitis and prescribed antibiotics. A few days later, I flew home on a red-eye flight and found him in bed in excruciating pain. I immediately took him to the emergency room, where they ran a series of tests. I will never forget when the doctor walked into the room to inform us that Neil had pancreatic cancer that had spread to other organs. They gave him 2-3 months to live.

At that moment, our world came crashing down around us. How does a 37-year-old man get diagnosed with terminal pancreatic cancer? The doctor admitted him to the hospital, and we met with an oncologist who prepared a plan of action and treatment. He was to start chemotherapy immediately following his discharge. Before leaving the hospital, Neil asked me, "Can you fix this? I will eat whatever you tell me to. I have to beat this cancer." So, we started on a vegetarian diet, and I scheduled him to meet with a naturopathic physician and acupuncturist to complement the therapy prescribed by his oncologist.

He did great in the initial months of chemotherapy. I made him a fruit smoothie every morning, followed by a 4-ounce glass of fresh wheatgrass. Lunch and dinner were plant-based meals with various fresh vegetables and sprouted grains. The naturopathic physician prescribed herbs, and we scheduled an acupuncture treatment any time this blood count started to fall below normal. He felt great and continued going to the gym and working every day. He lost a little weight, but despite everything happening internally, he appeared fantastic on the outside.

This new lifestyle was not easy. It took time and planning, but we had a reason to change our ways. Neil struggled emotionally but was determined to beat this diagnosis. Unfortunately, ten months after his pancreatic cancer diagnosis, Neil passed away on June 6, 2009.

I can't tell you how many times I relived those months asking myself why this happened to such a young man. What could we have done differently? Could we have caught it sooner had he gone to the doctor? Did the steroid use and growth hormones have anything to do with the diagnosis? Was it genetics? Why didn't we take the blood sugar issues more seriously? Why did we wait so long?

Most people wait to make lifestyle changes until a condition presents itself. Fortunately, many conditions can be managed and even reversed with diet, physical activity, and stress reduction. Heart disease is a perfect example of how diet and exercise can not only decrease the risk of disease but also manage and reverse symptoms associated with heart disease. Unfortunately, cancer is more challenging. Diet and exercise have been shown to help reduce the risk of cancer development, but diet and exercise alone are not sufficient once diagnosed. But with early detection and a combination of healthy lifestyle choices and the right medications or surgical interventions, cancer can be managed.

Yesterday, we discussed listening to your body. You must also listen to your body when something does not feel right. Is there something that concerns you? Are you avoiding the doctor? Why? How long will you keep the blinders on before you take charge and take control of your health? What frightens you to seek advice? You are reading this book because you want to change something in your life. So, what is stopping you from making a change?

Neil regretted that he lived life thinking that he was invincible. He wished that he had taken his health more seriously. No one expects a young adult to be diagnosed with a life-threatening disease. But it happens. More often than we want to acknowledge. Unfortunately, none of us is invincible, and we never truly know the root cause of an illness. Within ten years, I lost my mom and Neil to cancer. They were both so young. Was it their lifestyle or genetics? I will never know for certain. However, we do know that we can decrease our risks, and research has *proven* that diet, exercise, and stress reduction can reduce the incidence of disease.

What are you waiting for? The right time? There will never be *a* perfect time. You just need to do it. You need to be proactive. You *can* take control of your health. And today is the perfect day to do so. I feel that Neil's outcome could have been different had we been more proactive and understood the detriment of the lifestyle he chose to follow for so many years.

I have learned a precious lesson from losing my loved ones: I have a choice in every moment. I choose how to nourish my body and mind. I choose stress-free situations. I choose to go to bed early. I educate myself to make the best-informed decisions that will lead to my well-being. I respect my need for self-care. *You* have the same power. The choices you make each day can affect the likelihood of disease outcomes later in life. Will you take a proactive approach and start today? Not tomorrow. Today.

And, regarding my doctor's recommendation for a mastectomy and hysterectomy, I chose to find a new doctor. Instead, I choose to be proactive with routine screening, eating a balanced diet, alleviating stress by exercising daily, spending time with my family, and practicing self-care.

Here are healthy ideas you can do daily:

- Stay hydrated by drinking a glass of water when you wake up and throughout the day.
- Eat a colorful diet (fruits and veggies are very colorful).
- For every 50 minutes sitting down, get up and move or stretch for 5-10 minutes.
- Eat mindfully at each meal.
- Get plenty of rest and strive for at least 6-7 hours of sleep each night.
- Disconnect from emails, social media, and the computer in the evening.
- Do one type of physical activity daily: walking, biking, lifting weights, or stretching.
- Eat plant-based sources of lean protein such as beans, nuts, and seeds daily.
- Enjoy daily healthy fats such as avocados, fish, and olive oil.
- Exercise daily.
- Spend time doing things that make you happy.
- Laugh often.
- Get annual physicals.
- Listen to your body when something doesn't seem right.

Summary:

- Fifteen percent of diagnosed cases of disease, such as heart disease, diabetes, and cancer, are related to genetics. The remaining 85% of cases are due to lifestyle choices.

- Every day, you can choose to do something that can impact your risk of developing a disease.

- You have a choice in every moment.

- Factors you can control include the foods you eat, how physically active you are, how you react to stress, the environment in which you live and work, and how much sleep you get each night.

- There are some factors that we cannot change, such as our age, gender, and genetic makeup, but what we can change is our environment, which plays a role in genetic expression.

Achievable Actions:

- Choose 1-2 things you can do differently today that may impact your overall health. *If you are unsure what to choose, please pick items from my list of healthy ideas.*

Day 8

Do What You Love

I spent eight years attending yoga classes and not knowing what I was doing. I did yoga because yoga was the thing to do. Everyone was doing it. So, I struggled through the class and cursed through sun salutations, not understanding why I was putting myself through this hot, bendy workout I didn't love. But I kept going to class so I could say, "I do yoga all the time. Don't you?"

I will get to the point and say: ***don't do something you don't love.*** Ever. There are so many ways to be physically active; why do something you hate? You will never get anywhere and are more likely to give up if you force yourself to do something that someone else loves. Find what you love.

I love exercising, but yoga wasn't love at first backbend. My love for yoga did not happen until a friend took me to a studio called American Yoga. I went to that studio with great hesitation, mostly because my first experience with this particular yoga instructor was not great. It drove me crazy that she closed her eyes while she taught the class. I was frustrated that I couldn't grasp the poses – and forget trying to do a headstand. I did not understand the hype surrounding yoga and entered the studio with a negative mindset.

But I fell in love with yoga after my first class with this instructor. She was amazing, and I was hooked. She helped me to understand yoga on a deeper level and enhanced my practice. She taught me to do a headstand, amongst other things. Most importantly, I appreciated how yoga could be an intense workout but also a restorative practice for healing. All I had to do was listen to what my body needed in that moment. And that instructor has become one of my dearest friends.

I fell in love with yoga when I stopped being a follower.

I fell in love with yoga when I overcame my fears of feeling inadequate.

I fell in love with yoga when I started doing it for myself rather than because everyone else did.

I fell in love with yoga because it cleared the clutter in my mind.

I loved yoga so much that I earned my 200-hour yoga teaching certification, and for my Ph.D. dissertation, I conducted a research study demonstrating the benefits of yoga for breast cancer survivors. In many ways, yoga gave me a purpose. What purpose could you get from doing something you love?

On Day 1, I shared with you that I became a nutritionist to help others. I accomplished this goal through my education and being willing to explore outside of my comfort zone. I also mentioned that health goals will change as we move through life's experiences. My choices of physical activity have changed over the years based on my situation. During COVID, I stopped practicing yoga *for two years.* I shifted from yoga to working out using apps and then the gym when things re-opened. This will happen for you, too. And it is okay to make changes that suit you.

Before losing Neil to pancreatic cancer, I trained with a personal trainer. After his passing, I resumed my workouts with the trainer, but she had one stipulation. This stipulation shifted my mindset, and the outcome made me realize I had potential beyond my wildest expectations.

The one stipulation was that I had to train for a half-marathon. I laughed and told her she was crazy; she knew I hated to run. But I needed a distraction and desperately needed to escape the thoughts in my head. So, with great hesitation, I started running. Cursing all the way to the finish line. Ironically, the day of the half-marathon was my mom's birthday, and I dedicated that run to Neil while raising money for pancreatic research. I had a lot to celebrate that day.

Running became a way to clear my thoughts and strategize my day. I grew to love my morning runs. Most importantly, I loved how it made me feel. I felt accomplished. I felt fit. I was the most motivated I had ever been in my life. It was truly amazing. Interestingly, my first half-marathon was also my last half-marathon.

Yes, my *last* half-marathon. What changed? I did. I no longer needed to quiet the chatter in my head. I didn't have to run six miles to strategize my day. Life was getting easier for me. I met Rob, and I quickly fell in love. When love was the last thing I was looking for, love found me.

Today, I do what my body tells me to. When my hips feel tight, and my shoulders are stiff from sitting at my desk, I roll out my yoga mat. When I need to shake off my day, I lift weights. When I am tired and need some motivation, I jump on the Peloton. The best part is that Rob is right beside me. He makes me accountable, and we push each other daily to be better, stronger, and to never stay in our comfort zone. Working out with a partner is key. But it doesn't have to be someone you know. Group classes are a great way to work out with others. Energy is contagious, so put yourself in a position to receive energy and motivation from others. Group fitness is a great way to feel inspired; hey, you just may meet your new best friend.

The point is that throughout the past 20 years, I have both hated and loved exercise. At times, it felt pointless and something I had to do because everyone else was doing step aerobics. Today, I exercise because my body needs it. My mind needs it. And I love it. When you start exercising based on your body's needs, you will fall in love with it.

I want to point out that I did not *quit* running. I didn't *quit* yoga. I merely changed what I needed based on where I was in my life. I found what I love, and I am okay with trying new things and moving on from forms of exercise that no longer serve me. Running served a purpose for me when I needed it. I kept an open mind and have ever since. My wish for you is that you, too, can keep an open mind and try things that you never thought you could do, like running a half marathon.

I also encourage you to let go of things that don't serve you. Do you hate your gym? Find a new gym or an activity you can do outside of the gym. Don't stop working out because you had a bad experience. Instead, create a new experience. My yoga journey was quite the experience, leading me to self-fulfillment and an opportunity to work with a lovely group of women who kicked cancer's ass.

Be scared. Be adventurous. But most importantly, have fun. But, I must warn you of something important: *exercise has been shown to cause health and happiness*. Try it at your own risk. The results just may amaze you.

The benefits of exercise include:

- Improves sleep
- Reduces anxiety and depression
- Reduces stress
- Improves blood pressure

- Enhances brain health and memory
- Reduces the risk of heart disease, diabetes, and certain cancers
- Improves bone health
- Promotes weight loss
- Maintains a healthy body weight
- Improves digestion
- Reduces the risk of falls
- Enhances your mood
- Boosts energy
- Recharges your sex life
- Reduces chronic pain
- Increases your social activity

Exercise is defined as any movement that makes your muscles work and requires your body to burn calories. Thankfully, there are many types of physical activities, including running, walking, swimming, jogging, biking, stretching, playing outside with the kids, and dancing, to name a few. Being active has been shown to have long-term physical and mental benefits and may even help you live a longer, happier life. In contrast, a lack of regular exercise can significantly increase belly fat, which may increase the risk of type 2 diabetes, heart disease, and certain cancers.

Exercise increases the production of endorphins, which helps to alleviate pain, reduce stress, and improve well-being. Physical activity can increase brain sensitivity to the hormones serotonin and norepinephrine. Serotonin is the "feel good" hormone because it is associated with positive feelings and well-being and reduces anxiety, while norepinephrine can improve energy and alertness.

Do you have trouble sleeping at night? Then exercise is just what you need. Physical activity will increase your sleep drive, allowing you to fall asleep more quickly and improve sleep quality. The more physically active you are, the more rest you need. Since exercise reduces stress and anxiety, it promotes relaxation, which is key for a good night's rest. However, exercise can also energize you and may disrupt sleep cycles in some individuals. The good news is that exercising earlier in the day can easily fix this.

Since exercise releases endorphins, these chemicals boost brain activity and keep some people awake. Allow yourself at least 1 to 2 hours before bed to give yourself time to wind down. In addition, exercise will also increase your body's core temperature. The effect of exercise is like taking a shower in the morning to wake you up. Fortunately, the core body temperature starts to fall after about 30 to 90 minutes, and the decline helps to facilitate sleepiness.

Some people may avoid exercise due to age and health-related issues, especially those who experience chronic pain. For many years, the recommendation for treating chronic pain was to rest and avoid physical activity. However, recent studies show that exercise helps relieve chronic pain and improve life quality. Don't be afraid to move. I recommend working with trained health professionals and personal trainers to find what is right for your body. With the right exercise regimen, I guarantee you will feel improvements with aches and pains.

Lastly, as people age, they tend to lose muscle mass and function, which can lead to an increased risk of injury and falls. And when I say "as people age," I am not referring to your 60s and 70s. No, ma'am, you will begin to see the signs of aging in your 30s if you do not care for yourself. The best way to maintain muscle mass is to remain active throughout life. And it is never too late to start.

In addition to improving muscle mass, physical activity is especially important in older adults since aging can promote changes in brain structure and function. Exercise has been shown to improve mental function and reduce brain changes that can contribute to cognitive disorders like Alzheimer's disease and dementia.

If all of this information is insufficient to convince you to exercise, then you may be interested to know that exercise has been proven to boost sex drive. Regular exercise can strengthen the heart, improve blood circulation, and enhance flexibility, all promoting a healthy sex life. So, there you have it, folks. Jump on that treadmill.

The great news is that it doesn't take much movement to make a big difference in your health. According to the Physical Activity Guidelines for Americans issued by the U.S. Department of Health and Human Services, adults need 150 minutes of moderate-intensity aerobic activity each week plus two days of muscle-strengthening activity. That might sound like a lot, but you don't have to do it all simultaneously. It could be 30 minutes a day, 5 days a week. You can spread your activity out during the week and break it up into smaller chunks of time. Keep in mind these recommendations are the minimum requirements. As you progress and get stronger, I encourage you to exercise daily.

Today, I want you to explore different options and find a new exercise you want to try. You can browse the web for local classes, community activities, dance lessons, and gyms in your area. Feel free to visit www.tammyfogarty.com and read about my favorite apps and trainers that offer free routines you can do from home, outside, or at your gym. When planning to try something new, consider the following:

- Choose an exercise you will enjoy.
- Choose options that fit your lifestyle.
- Consider joining a class. The social interaction is motivating.

- Choose an exercise that can become part of your daily routine.
- Choose something that accommodates physical or health concerns.
- Choose a partner to exercise with you. Your partner can be non-human; walking the dog is exercise for you and your pup.

Tomorrow, I will provide tips so that you can prioritize physical activity in your normal daily routine.

Summary:

- You are more likely to give up exercising if you force yourself to do something that someone else loves. Find what you love.

- Exercise is any movement that makes your muscles work and requires your body to burn calories.

- There are many types of physical activity, including running, walking, swimming, jogging, biking, stretching, playing outside with the kids, and dancing, to name a few.

- Exercise can increase the production of endorphins, which helps to alleviate pain, reduce stress, and improve your well-being.

- Activity increases your sleep drive, allowing you to fall asleep more quickly and improving sleep quality.

- Exercise helps relieve chronic pain and improve quality of life.

- The best way to maintain muscle mass is to remain active throughout life

- Exercise has been proven to boost sex drive.

Achievable Actions:

- Explore different types of activity.
- Try one new exercise today.
- Download my free exercise journal at www.tammyfogarty.com.

Day 9

Prioritize Physical Activity

How did it go yesterday? Did you try something new? If not, okay, then TODAY is the day! But to do this, you must not think of exercising as something you *have to* do. Exercise is not a chore. It is an opportunity to move your body, exceed your limitations, and feel physically and mentally good. You are one burpee away from a good time. Just kidding, they are not a good time. I hate burpees. They make me want to puke, but I still do them. Hey, why don't you give them a try today?

Instead of perceiving exercise as a chore, I want you to think of yourself as an athlete, a runner, a yogi, or a healthy person. Whoever you would like to be. When in doubt about trying something new, think of a person who *would* try it and ask yourself, "What would that person do?" and then do it! Today, you are one exercise closer to a good mood, a stronger body, and getting a full night's rest.

Physical activity supports physical and mental health and is one of the most important things you can do for your health. Health benefits start immediately after exercising, and even short episodes of physical activity are beneficial. Unfortunately, about half of all American adults, that's 117 million people, have one or more *preventable* chronic diseases. Seven of the ten most common chronic diseases are positively influenced by regular physical activity. Yet nearly 80 percent of adults do not meet the guidelines for both aerobic and strength-building activity. Eighty percent! That's a lot of people not exercising.

This lack of physical activity is linked to approximately $120 billion in annual healthcare costs and about 10 percent of premature deaths. Therefore, the US Department of Health and Human Services composed a committee of researchers in the fields of physical activity, health, and medicine to create the Physical Activity Guidelines for Americans. Here are what the guidelines say:

For substantial health benefits, healthy adults should:

- Do at least 150 minutes (2 hours and 30 minutes) to 300 minutes (5 hours) a week of moderate-intensity or 75 minutes (1 hour and 15 minutes) to 150 minutes (2 hours and 30 minutes) a week of vigorous-intensity aerobic physical activity, or an equivalent combination of moderate- and vigorous-intensity aerobic activity.

- Preferably, aerobic activity should be spread throughout the week.

Here are examples of light, moderate, and vigorous physical activities:

- Light: Walking slowly, sitting at the computer, standing light work such as cooking or washing dishes.

- Moderate: Brisk walking, mowing the lawn, vacuuming, cycling 10-12 mph

- Vigorous: Hiking, jogging/running at 6 mph, shoveling, cycling 14-16 mph, soccer, basketball

There are two categories of exercise: aerobic and anaerobic:

Aerobic exercise can reduce the risk of diseases, such as heart disease, diabetes, and cancer, and is known as cardiovascular training or "cardio." Cardio training requires oxygen; therefore, your breathing and heart rate increase for a sustained period of time. Examples of aerobic activities include swimming laps, running, cycling, dancing, cross-country skiing, stair climbing, or rowing.

Benefits of aerobic activity include:

- may promote weight loss
- lowers blood pressure
- may reduce fatigue during exercise by increasing stamina
- strengthens your heart and lungs to boost cardiorespiratory fitness
- enhances your mood
- improves the quality of life

It is important to start slowly with any new workout routine and work up gradually to reduce your risk of an injury. For example, start walking for 5 minutes, and add 5 minutes daily until you're up to a 30-minute brisk walk.

Anaerobic exercise can be beneficial if you're looking to build muscle or lose weight. Anaerobic exercise involves quick bursts of energy performed at maximum effort for a short time. Anaerobic activity includes jumping, sprinting, weightlifting, and high-intensity interval training.

Benefits of anaerobic activity include:

- strengthens bones and builds bone density
- burns fat
- builds muscle

- increases stamina for daily activities like dancing or playing with the kids

Both aerobic and anaerobic exercise can benefit everyone. But first, please consult with your doctor for approval if you've been inactive for a long time or live with a chronic condition. A certified fitness professional, Physical Therapist, or Athletic Trainer can help you create a suitable workout based on your medical history and health goals.

To help make sense of the exercise guidelines, here are examples of incorporating aerobic, anaerobic, and strength training.

Option 1: Moderate Intensity Aerobic Activity

A brisk walk for 30 minutes, five days a week **and** muscle-strengthening activities on two or more days a week that work all major muscle groups (legs, hips, back, abdomen, chest, shoulders, and arms).

Option 2: Vigorous Intensity Aerobic Activity

A 25-minute run or jog three days a week **and** muscle-strengthening activities on two or more days a week that work all major muscle groups (legs, hips, back, abdomen, chest, shoulders, and arms).

Option 3: Mix of Moderate and Vigorous Intensity Aerobic Activity

A 30-minute cycle three days a week **and** a 25-minute jog one day per week **and** two or more days a week that work all major muscle groups (legs, hips, back, abdomen, chest, shoulders, and arms).

Tips to Stay Motivated:

- Choose something you enjoy doing.
    - One reason people find that their exercise program falls by the wayside is boredom. If you enjoy going for a walk, turn it into a daily routine and steadily increase your pace and how far you walk. Try exercising at home if you don't enjoy going to the gym. Do something fun, such as dancing or riding bikes with the kids. Continually try new activities to keep yourself interested and motivated.

- Choose more than one type of exercise.
    - Include a combination of aerobic and anaerobic activities to spice up your workout. Sticking to the same routine creates monotony and reduces motivation. Instead, add a variety of exercises that work different muscles on different days. This technique will help reduce the risk of injury and eliminate boredom.

- Vary the intensity of your workout.
    - Some days, you will come out guns blazing; other days, you may be dragging butt. It is good to vary the intensity of your workout to allow for recovery from the days you go all out. For example, restorative yoga to open and stretch your hip flexors will feel great after a few days of cycling or running. Listen to your body; it will tell you what it needs.

- Join a class.
    - I never really kick my butt when I exercise, so I love classes that push me beyond my expectations and give me a good ass-kicking. Social interaction is a great motivator and creates a sense of community.

- Exercise with a partner.
    - Maintaining the motivation to exercise regularly is challenging for many people. Including a partner in your new-found exercise interest might include booking a court for weekly social pickleball, riding bikes with the kids after dinner, or arranging to walk each morning with a nearby friend.

- Schedule exercise.
    - This may sound silly, but schedule time for exercise, just as you would schedule an appointment. Setting aside time each day can help turn regular exercise into a habit, like grabbing coffee in the morning. And, don't cancel on yourself! Keep your appointment.

Summary:

- Exercise is not a chore. It is an opportunity to exceed your limitations and feel physically and mentally good.

- Physical activity supports physical and mental health and is one of the most important things you can do for your health.

- Health benefits start immediately after exercising, and even short episodes of physical activity are beneficial.

- Aerobic exercise can reduce the risk of diseases, such as heart disease, diabetes, and cancer, and is known as cardiovascular training or "cardio."

- Anaerobic exercise can be beneficial if you're looking to build muscle or lose weight.

- A certified fitness professional, Physical Therapist, or Athletic Trainer can help you create a suitable workout based on your medical history and health goals.

Achievable Actions:

- Create an exercise plan for the week.
- Schedule time in your calendar to exercise.
- Visit www.tammyfogarty.com to download the Exercise Journal.

Day 10

Set a Goal. Or Don't. Choose What Works for You.

For the past nine days, you have determined what healthy means; you have ditched the diet mindset, are mindfully eating fiber-rich carbs, healthy fats, and lean protein, and have scheduled your workouts. Now, let's create a PACT to get things done.

Have you ever had a goal? The definition of a goal is *the object of a person's ambition or effort, an aim or desired result.* Most of us start the new year with the best intentions to work out, eat healthy, and go to bed early. But, after a few weeks, the novelty wears off, and we instead choose to binge the newest series on Netflix rather than go to the gym or order takeout. We promise to do better tomorrow, next week, or next month. Or you may throw in the towel and make it next year's resolution.

Imagine yourself a year from now, having tried the same goal and being in the same spot as when you started. Do you feel trapped by your goals? Do you feel like a failure because you haven't met your goals? Do you feel trapped by the goals you created? You're not alone. Personally, I am not a fan of goals and prefer the term "desired result." After all, the subtitle of this book is *A Simple Guide to Reaching Your Health Goals and Making Better Choices in the Moment.* Today, you will do just that.

The first issue with goal setting is related to how the brain works. As a nutritionist, I help people change their eating patterns to promote health or manage an illness. For example, a person diagnosed with diabetes must follow a specific meal pattern to manage blood glucose levels. I develop specific goals that promote behavioral change, encouraging healthy eating patterns and exercise. However, it is not uncommon for clients to report they do not "feel good" after making these changes.

Theoretically, this makes no sense because eating a healthy, balanced diet should make them feel *better*. Let me ask you, have you ever felt bad after eating a certain food? Sure, we all have. However, I have found that people get used to feeling "bad." If you consistently consume junky foods, you get comfortable with feeling like junk. And feeling junky will bring you comfort. Any shift in the diet, such as adding fresh fruit and vegetables, can make a person feel different and uncomfortable.

This is where the brain works protectively and resists change. The brain is wired to seek rewards and avoid pain or discomfort, including fear. When fear of failure is present, there is a desire to return to known, comfortable behaviors or to resume consuming junk foods and a sedentary lifestyle. That is exactly what happens to most people when they start working out or completely change their diet. The reaction is to abort mission and stop doing the things that make you feel bad, even though these changes are good for you.

However, this long, uncomfortable tunnel has a light at the end. Over time, your body will become accustomed to eating healthy foods, exercising, and feeling good. So, give yourself some time and stick with it. Your new routine will eventually become your new normal. You will also notice that being sedentary and eating junky food doesn't feel good at all.

The second problem with goal setting is that goals create an ideal image of perfection, which can activate judgmental thinking of "I should be this way." We often think we are failures or not good enough if we do not meet a goal. Therefore, setting big, lofty goals may not be the best plan of action when you want to create long-term, healthy changes.

Now, this doesn't mean you stop achieving things. It means you stop limiting yourself with unrealistic goals. While you might desire to run a marathon, the goal of doing so may feel overwhelming when you lace up your running shoes for the first time. But what if the goal was to run for 10 minutes daily?

Focusing on smaller goals to achieve the grand prize is the strategy behind setting micro-goals. Rather than setting a big goal, like running a marathon, think of the smallest action you could achieve daily. Celebrating the completion of small accomplishments allows you to feel good about yourself every day. This is known as the psychology of small wins, and we will focus on how doing small things can equate to BIG rewards.

Micro-goals are small, achievable goals that you can do in under 10 minutes daily. And we all have 10 minutes to do something good for ourselves. Done with intention, completing a micro-goal each day is a form of continuous improvement that helps us get a little better each day. James Clear, the author of *Atomic Habits*, describes "the power of tiny gains." He explains that "incremental improvement adds up, considering the compounding gains of getting just 1% better daily." Basically, if you can get 1% better each day for one year, you'll end up thirty-seven times better by the time you are done. What starts as a small win can accumulate into something much more.

On Day 1, I asked you to define what health means to you and a goal you will work on. Today, you will work on creating micro-goals that will empower you to develop healthy habits. Here is how it works:

BIG GOALS	MICRO-GOALS
Get healthy	Eat one piece of fruit each day
Get fit	Walk around the block each morning
Lose weight	Eat a salad at dinner each day
Get organized	Make the bed when you get up

A micro-goal shifts the focus from what you hope to achieve in the future to actions you can achieve right now. Micro-goals are the plan that allows you to execute a result. At the end of each day, I provide you with a list of achievable actions. By choosing to follow through with an achievable action, you are already familiar with micro-goals. And by completing micro-goals daily, you will create habits that will stick with you long-term.

The best part of achieving micro-goals is that it will push you to do more. For example, your stroll around the block can transform into a jog around the neighborhood. Eating a salad with dinner will encourage you to eat vegetables throughout the day. And as you celebrate your small wins daily, you will feel less overwhelmed about reaching the larger goal. You will get there. Just give yourself time and celebrate the small wins.

Please realize that weight gain does not happen overnight, so you cannot expect immediate weight loss. Heart disease doesn't appear one day; it results from years of unhealthy habits and takes time to reverse the damage. In reality, all things take time. You must respect that and give yourself the time you need. Small changes will promote habits that produce desirable results. What small changes can you make today?

I understand that some people need direction and guidance to make changes. Therefore, I will share a second strategy for those needing a bit more structure and a plan. PACT is a goal-setting technique and stands for Purposeful, Actionable, Continuous, and Trackable. I like to share this strategy because it focuses on taking action, allows you to reassess, and encourages continuous progress.

Here are the four elements of PACT and how they can help you achieve your goals:

Purposeful

A "Purposeful" effort represents a meaning and the passion that drives you toward achieving the goal. Your goal must have a purpose and fulfill a need or want. Sticking to your goal will be much harder if you don't care. When a goal is aligned with your passions and objectives, you feel motivated and are more likely to achieve desired results.

Actionable

Being "Actionable" means making efforts to change the things within your reach that you can control now instead of focusing on distant outcomes. Live in the moment. It's about shifting your mindset from what may happen in the future to what is within your reach now and taking action today rather than overplanning for tomorrow.

Continuous

The actions you take toward your goal must be simple and repeatable. With the "Continuous" pursuit of repeatable and straightforward routines, we can avoid "choice paralysis." That's when there are so many options that you spend more time researching all the different things you could do rather than making progress toward your goal immediately.

The good thing about continuous goals is their flexibility. You can adapt your approach as you learn more about your goal and the changes within yourself. On Day 8, I shared with you how the types of physical activities I engaged in have changed over the years based on what I needed at the moment. The goal was to keep exercising, but I had the flexibility to change the type of exercise to suit my needs. The same rings true with any healthy habit you want to achieve. Focus on continuous improvement rather than reaching a supposed end goal. Progress over perfection. Feel free to experiment through continuous actions, and then measure success through your effort and progress.

Trackable

Being able to track accomplishments can positively impact mental health and wellness as it pertains to a sense of accomplishment based on effort and progress. I support a "yes" or "no" approach to goal tracking. Have you done the thing or not? Did you eat fruit today? Did you walk around the block? Yes or no? This makes your progress very easy to track rather than the mundane task of tracking how many servings of fruit you ate or miles you walked.

For example, your micro-goal is to eat fruit daily. Did you do it? Yes. Fantastic! Check it off your list and move on. Some may be skeptical and say this is too easy, and people can cheat by checking yes, even if only one grape was consumed. My friend, it is your choice not to do what you set out to do. I am not the fruit police. You know if you are cutting corners and not doing the work. I can't help you with that. No one can. Only you can make that call, do what you must, and eat the friggin' fruit. And guess what? One grape is better than no grapes. Additionally, if you are avoiding fruit, perhaps it is not the goal for you, and you need to refer back to the previous section on continuous changes.

Ultimately, you know what will work for you. For some people, setting a defined goal with an action plan is necessary. For others, taking smaller steps and living in the moment is a more realistic approach. Today, we discussed two strategies: PACT and micro-goals. PACT goals are designed to get you started right now. What action do you want to take that will help you improve? Micro-goals are small, achievable goals you can do in under 10 minutes every day. I suggest starting with one or two micro-goals, building upon them as you go. If you need more structure and a defined plan, move on to create a PACT goal. Whatever your strategy may be, just start. Start working towards whatever makes you happy and comfortable within yourself. I will introduce you to strategies to improve your health and well-being in the upcoming days. Feel free to create micro-goals to incorporate these changes into your daily routine.

Please visit *www.tammyfogarty.com* to download the PACT template and micro-goals worksheet.

Summary:

- The brain is wired to seek rewards and avoid pain or discomfort, including fear.

- Stop limiting yourself with unrealistic goals.

- Rather than setting a big goal, think of the smallest action you could take each day to accomplish what you ultimately want.

- Micro-goals are small, achievable goals that you can do in under 10 minutes daily.

- A small win can accumulate into something much more.

- PACT is a goal-setting technique and stands for Purposeful, Actionable, Continuous, and Trackable.

Achievable Actions:

- Identify a goal or desired result (get fit, lose weight, reduce stress).
- Establish 1-2 micro-goals using the Micro-Goal worksheet.
- Create your PACT goal using the PACT template.

Day 11

Overcome Challenges

Yesterday, you identified a desired result (goal) and 1-2 micro-goals to work on daily. Today I want to focus on the obstacles that may get in the way and how to devise a plan to jump over obstacles before they interfere with your goal.

Most of my clients' nutrition counseling is related to weight loss and fitness. The plan is to get healthy by losing weight and getting into shape. However, "something" always gets in the way of my clients achieving their goals. From the start, we discuss the "things" that can become an obstacle and brainstorm ways to avoid them. Common obstacles that get in the way of weight loss include:

- I don't have time to prepare meals
- I don't have time to go to the grocery store
- My kids won't eat healthy food
- Healthy foods are boring/taste bad
- I don't know how to cook
- It is so hard to eat healthy during the holidays
- I love to go out with my friends
- I can't give up my wine at night
- I don't know what to order at a restaurant

- I wish I had someone to do this diet with
- I need someone to tell me what to eat
- My significant other does not support my attempts to lose weight

Any of these sound familiar? How about obstacles related to exercising:

- I am too tired
- I am stressed out
- I don't have time to get to the gym
- I don't know what to do at the gym
- I hate the freakin' gym
- I am uncomfortable being around all those fit people
- My back (knees, legs, etc.) hurts
- I have to take my kids to their extracurricular activities and don't have time to get to the gym
- I wish I had someone who would go to the gym with me
- My significant other does not support my attempts to work out

Sound familiar? Everyone can relate to these challenges. They are real and create an obstacle to successful change. In addition, change is a process that we don't love and need to become comfortable with. If you are a parent, think of when your child says they don't like to do something at school, or perhaps they don't want to participate in a sport at school because the other kids are better than they are. What advice do you give your child?

Most likely, you encourage them to give it a try. You motivate them to do it. Why not do the same for yourself? Take the advice that you would offer your kid(s). Get out of your comfort zone, be okay with being uncomfortable, and find solutions to make it work. You would do the same for your kids. And I can promise you this; you will not regret it.

Have you experienced any of the following scenarios?

- Sitting on the couch watching TV after work because you are tired, so going to the gym may seem daunting. You will go tomorrow.

- You had a stressful day, so you grab your favorite comfort food and promise you will eat healthy tomorrow.

- The kids all want different things for dinner, so it is easier to run through the drive-thru so they can pick what they want.

- You make time for everyone else in the house, so there is little time for you at the end of the day.

- Your family makes you feel guilty because you have changed, which is now affecting them.

- Your plan to get healthy is straining your friendship(s) because you'd rather go to the gym and prepare a healthy meal at home than meet for drinks at happy hour.

There will always be something to interfere with your plans. ALWAYS. I mention throughout this book that you have a choice in every moment. I also want you to understand that the difference between an obstacle and an opportunity is your mindset. You can allow the obstacle to get in your way or you can take the opportunity to overcome any obstacle that comes your way. You get to choose your mindset. For example, you may feel you are missing out on spending time with your friends by skipping happy hour. Let's flip the script. You can still spend time with your friends and choose to skip the wine.

Here is another common scenario: you feel that your family is not supportive, and you are missing out on eating the foods you and your family love. Change your mindset and find a healthy version of your family's favorite recipe. You can choose to include them by preparing a family meal together. Make it a family affair!

Lastly, you want to spend less time on social media but don't want to miss out on good posts. Instead, limit your time on social media and use the time to prepare a healthy meal. Your reward will be to browse social media after your delicious dinner and maybe even an evening walk.

Be your own driving force. I can't do this for you, and neither will anyone else. I can give you advice, but *you* have to want it, and *you* have to do it. So, let's brainstorm ideas so you can tackle obstacles head-on.

Is your to-do list longer than the hours of the day? The greatest obstacle for most people is time. I would love a few more hours each day, but we must work with what we have. The best way to find more time is to determine what you are currently doing with your time. And yes, this is a time-consuming task that will be worth your time. Trust me.

I want you to track what you do throughout the day by recording activities. Record your activities from the moment you wake up to when you lie down to sleep. Here is an example:

7:00 am: Wake up and take a shower

7:15 am: Get the kids up so they can get ready for school

7:30 am: Give the kids breakfast and start making their lunches

7:45 am: Finish getting ready for work

8:30 am: Drop kids off at school

9:00 am: Arrive at work

12:00 pm: Lunch at a restaurant with your co-workers

5:00 pm: Get the kids from aftercare

5:30 pm: Get the kids to soccer practice

6:30 pm: Round up the kids and take them to Chick-fil-A

7:00 pm: Kids work on homework while parents relax watching TV

8:00 pm: Get the kids ready for bed

9:00 pm: Kids are in bed; browse through social media while watching Netflix

11:00 pm: Go to bed

In this example, there is not much time to go grocery shopping, let alone cook a meal, followed by a workout at the gym. Or is there? Can you do the following things to help free up time during the day?

- Get up an hour earlier?
- Go for a walk in the morning?
- Place a grocery store delivery, such as Instacart, during your lunch hour and plan for it to be delivered around the time you get home?
- In the evening, can you take 20 minutes to prepare lunch for the next day for you and the kids?
- After you make those lunches, do you have another 15 minutes to prepare breakfast for the next morning, such as overnight oats, cut-up fruit, or breakfast burritos that can be warmed up?
- Can you go to bed 30 minutes earlier so a 6:00 a.m. wake-up call doesn't feel so early?
- When you make dinner, can you make extra to have leftovers for lunch?

Here is what your day could look like.

6:00 am: Get up and go for a 30-minute brisk walk or a jog

6:45 am: Get ready for work

7:00 am: Wake up the kids so they can get ready

7:30 am: Have the breakfast you prepared the night before and enjoy time with the kids rather than rushing out the door for school

8:30 am: Drop the kids off

9:00 am: Fill your water bottle and start your work day

12:00 pm: Unwrap the delicious lunch that you prepared the night before and take a few minutes to browse the web to find a recipe the whole family will love. Then, take 10 minutes to order groceries to be delivered at 6:15.

5:00 pm: Pick up the kids.

5:30 pm: Take the kiddos to their extracurricular activities.

6:30 pm: Make dinner with your family. Involve the kids. They will be more willing to try new foods if they are involved.

7:30 pm: Kids wrap up homework, and you can take dinner leftovers and incorporate them into lunch for the next day. Prep a simple breakfast for the next day.

8:00 pm: Get the kids ready for bed.

9:00 pm: Roll out a yoga mat and do some light stretches as you wind down for bed.

9:30 pm: Crawl into bed with a book to help prepare you for sleep.

These two scenarios are not much different. The kids still need breakfast, a ride to school, afterschool activities, dinner, and time to unwind from the day. However, in the second scenario, you:

- Have quality time with your kids enjoying breakfast prepared the night before
- Enjoy a healthy lunch using leftovers from dinner. Preparing lunch also reduces the excess calories you would likely consume while eating at a restaurant.
- Arrange to have groceries delivered so that you can prepare a meal with your family following after-school activities.
- Go to bed a little earlier so that you wake feeling refreshed and ready for your morning walk.

Making small changes can impact your day significantly. But the key is to *keep things simple.* Here are some examples:

- Prepping breakfast and lunch for the next day can be time-consuming, so don't attempt to prepare gourmet meals during the week. Instead, make a simple salad or sandwich for lunch and add fresh fruit to your overnight oats.

- Don't complicate your day by expecting that you can fit in a two-hour workout. Do short, effective workouts throughout the day. I lift light weights during Zoom meetings, jump on the spin bike for 20 minutes, and do a quick 30-minute high-intensity workout with my husband after work.

- Grilled chicken and a salad go a long way. A hearty bowl of chili is an excellent source of fiber, protein, and healthy fat. Choose recipes that are easy and don't require much prep time. One-pot suppers are the best! And always make a little extra for lunch the next day.

Here are some additional tips to overcome the most common challenges:

- My kids won't eat healthy food.

- Create a Pinterest account and ask them to choose one meal they want to make that week. Of course, you will need to set parameters, such as each meal should include one vegetable, but giving the kiddos the option to choose goes a long way. And, if they help prepare a meal, they are more likely to eat it.

- What do you do if the kids don't want to eat healthy foods? Start small. Ask your kids to create micro-goals. For example, one micro-goal is to eat one serving of a vegetable at dinner and one piece of fruit every day.

- Get the kids involved. Don't expect that everyone in your family is on board with your goals. Most likely, they are not okay with changing their diet and will resist eating new foods. So, get them involved. Studies show that when kids take part in food preparation, they are more likely to eat the foods they make.

- Healthy foods are boring/taste bad.
    - I call bullshit on this one! If you use this excuse, you don't want to eat salad. And guess what? No one says you have to eat salad to be healthy. I have come across some pretty unhealthy salads. And let's be honest, not all healthy foods taste bad. Instead, try new things and learn to prepare foods differently. Experiment with fresh herbs. Make cooking fun by scheduling a family cooking class.

- It is so hard to eat healthy during the holidays.
    - Be the person who brings a healthy side dish. Just because it is the holidays doesn't mean that everything is unhealthy. Plenty of options on a holiday table aren't terrible for you. Plan to eat

more of the healthier options and less of the unhealthy ones. Better yet, the holidays are the perfect time to practice Mindful Eating. No one says you can't enjoy all the Thanksgiving fixings; just eat smaller portions. Lastly, don't go to the party hungry. Eat a healthy meal or snack before you arrive so you don't overindulge. An apple is small but a mighty nutrient-dense food. It will fill you up so you don't overeat during your meal. Most importantly, it's the holidays, so enjoy yourself. This is not the time to go on a diet.

- I don't know what to order at a restaurant.
    - Take a peek at the menu online and choose a healthy option. There is no need to peruse through the menu once you get there; this will only create the temptation to order something different. Stick with your choice and enjoy it! You can look ahead to Day 20 if you want more tips for dining out.

Summary:

- There will always be "something" that gets in the way of my clients achieving a goal.

- Have a plan to overcome challenges that threaten your success.

- Change is a process that we don't love but need to become comfortable with.

- Making small changes can impact your day significantly.

- Keep it simple.

Achievable Actions:

- Identify at least 1-2 obstacles that may interfere with your goal.

- Determine how you will overcome each obstacle. Make sure to write out your plan to prepare when the time comes.

- Please visit www.tammyfogarty.com and download the PACT or micro-goals worksheet. There is a place for you to plan for potential obstacles.

Day 12

Rethink Your Drink

How much water should you drink each day? This is such a simple question with no easy answer. Water recommendations do not fit into a one-size-fits-all category, and several factors affect how much we need. Let's start by discussing why we need water so you can determine how much is sufficient.

Water is an essential nutrient, and optimal hydration is key to good health. Water accounts for approximately 60% of an adult's body weight, and blood plasma is comprised of about 90% water. We must drink sufficient water to prevent dehydration and restore fluids lost through metabolism, breathing, sweating, urination, and bowel movements.

Water helps to maintain body temperature and will keep you from overheating. In addition, water lubricates the joints and tissues, maintains healthy skin, is necessary for proper digestion, and prevents constipation and kidney stones. Water is the best option to quench your thirst and hydrate your body. Lastly, water is the perfect zero-calorie beverage.

Daily total water intake is the amount consumed from foods, drinking water, and other beverages. The required daily varies by age, sex, pregnancy, and breastfeeding status. Most of your fluid needs are met via water and other beverages, but it is important to remember that foods with high water content, such as fruits and vegetables, are also a way to hydrate the body.

Most of us drink fluids with meals, but sometimes we drink based on how much we think we should drink. One of the most familiar sayings is to aim for "8 glasses a day," but this may not be appropriate for every person. How much fluid does the average healthy adult need? The U.S. National Academies of Sciences, Engineering, and Medicine determined that an adequate daily fluid intake is:

- About 15.5 cups (3.7 liters or 124 fluid ounces) a day for men
- About 11.5 cups (2.7 liters or 92 fluid ounces) a day for women

These recommendations include fluids from water, other beverages, and food. About 20% of daily fluid intake usually comes from food, and the remaining 80% comes from water and beverages. For some people, fewer than eight cups a day might be enough. But other people might need more.

Most healthy people can stay hydrated by drinking water and other fluids whenever thirsty. Thirst is the first sign that you need to drink water and may sometimes indicate mild dehydration. You might need to modify your total fluid intake based on several factors:

- **Exercise.** Sweat equates to water loss. The more you sweat, the more water you must drink. Drinking water before, during, and after a workout is important.

- **Environment.** I live in hot, steamy South Florida, so being sweaty is normal, and that is why you see many Floridians carrying a water bottle with them. If your state has hot or humid weather, you need extra fluids. High altitudes can cause dehydration, even when it is cold. Check in with yourself and drink water, especially when you feel thirsty.

- **Overall health.** You will lose bodily fluids due to a fever, vomiting, or diarrhea. Other conditions requiring increased fluid intake include constipation, bladder infections, and urinary tract stones. Stay hydrated and follow your doctor's recommendations related to oral rehydration solutions.

- **Pregnancy and breastfeeding.** If you are pregnant or breastfeeding, you will need additional fluids to keep mom and baby hydrated.

I enjoy drinking water, but most people prefer a flavorful beverage. Here are some great alternatives to good ol' water:

- **Add fruit.** Lemons, limes, and oranges are the most common, but don't be afraid to experiment with berries, cucumber, and watermelon. Herbs, such as mint and rosemary, also are delicious options.

- **Add some bubbles.** I love sparkling water, especially with lemon and mint. I drink it all day. I prefer to make my sparkling water using a carbonation machine, but stores carry a variety of flavored sparkling water you can enjoy.

- **Opt for coconut water.** Coconut water is a great option and has a mild, nutty flavor. Coconut water is also a great option after exercise to replenish sodium and potassium after a sweaty workout. And, if you want to get fancy, get coconut water with pulp. It's delicious and good for you.

- **Fresh pressed juice.** I love fresh juice. It contains vitamins and antioxidants and provides fructose if you need a little energy boost. Remember that an eight-ounce glass of juice contains approximately 115 calories and 30 grams of sugar. If you want the juice, but not all the calories and sugar, try a combination of half juice and half sparkling or plain water.

- **Iced Tea.** Iced tea is a great alternative to water and can give you a boost of antioxidants, depending on the type of tea. I prefer to brew herbal tea and love the variety of mint, berry, and green teas found in grocery stores. Get creative by adding mint and fresh raspberries to your iced tea, or make infused ice by adding fruit or herbs to your ice tray for a super fun drink.

Many of us are busy, and drinking water throughout the day is not at the top of the priority list. But it should be! If you don't drink throughout the day, here are some tips to keep you hydrated:

- **Find a cool cup.** Or as I call it, a feel-good mug. You are more likely to drink from a cup you like. So, find one that you LOVE and that makes you feel good when drinking from it. This cup will become your adult version of that special soft blanket you carried around as a child. I love insulated cups, such as Yeti, to keep my water cold all day. I even have a favorite smoothie cup. Find your favorite cup and drink up!

- **Grab a straw.** You will consume more if you drink from a straw. There is one downside of using straws – for some people, it can make you gassy and cause you to burp. So, if this is happening to you, ditch the straw and opt for a cool lid. Yeti cups come with cool lids, so you may want to make the investment and be part of the cool drinking club.

- **Carry it with you.** I carry a bottle of water everywhere: to the gym, in the car while running errands, while traveling, on the coffee table while watching television, and on my desk while working. You will drink more water, or the beverage of your choice, if it is readily available. Remember, out of sight, out of mind. Keep water in your sightline so you remember to drink throughout the day.

Summary:

- Water is essential and required for optimal hydration. Water is a key component of good health.

- Water helps to maintain body temperature and will keep you from overheating.

- Water is the best option to quench your thirst and hydrate your body.

Achievable Actions:

- Get cozy with your new cup. Find something that you like to drink out of.

- Carry a water bottle or your favorite new cup to remind you to drink.

- Get fancy by adding fruit and herbs to your water or create infused ice cubes.

Day 13

Out of Sight, Out of Mind

I love walking into a restaurant and seeing what the chefs are cooking. One of my favorite restaurants has the kitchen smack dab in your face when you walk through the door. At certain times of the year, they make grilled artichokes. Because I see the delicious artichokes when I walk in, it is the first thing I order.

Open-concept kitchens are designed to trigger the appetite when guests walk through the door. We truly eat with our eyes, especially with a little help from a hormone called ghrelin. Ghrelin is produced in the stomach and triggers appetite by acting on a region in your brain known for controlling the amount of food you eat. When you see food, ghrelin is released into the bloodstream, resulting in a spike in your appetite, signaling you to eat.

Even the smell of food sends signals throughout the body that we are ready to eat as soon as we catch a glimpse, or a good whiff, of food. The same happens in your home. The foods we see first are the most consumed. Think about when you open the refrigerator; what do you reach for? Usually, it is something easy to make or food you can grab and go. Unfortunately, quick and easy doesn't always equate to a healthy snack.

I get it; we are always on the move, so we need foods that are convenient. And who doesn't love a sweet and salty snack? However, we tend to snack the most when we are tired – too tired to prepare something healthy or cut up the giant watermelon staring at you from the back of the refrigerator. Chips are salty, delicious, and easy. Cutting down a watermelon takes some work. But, if you plan ahead and purchase pre-cut fruits and veggies, or do it yourself when you are feeling energized, the healthy snack is just as convenient as the unhealthy one. Seriously, it is just as easy to grab an apple as it is to grab a cookie. It's all about making a healthy choice in the moment.

The good news is that you have a choice of which foods you put on display. Today, your achievable action is to put the foods you would like to eat more of right in front of you. I want it to hit you in the face each time you open the refrigerator. Or, place a bowl of grapes on the counter so they can call your name each time you walk by. If you see it, you are more likely to eat it.

For example, I love veggies and usually eat them with each meal. I love fruit, too, but it is not something I reach for when I need a snack. Unfortunately, my refrigerator has been referred to as the fruit graveyard since many a fruit has rotted away while tucked in produce drawers. Therefore, I have to remind myself to eat fruit, and I do so by placing bowls of beautiful fruit in plain view. I also make it a point to cut up fruit and vegetables so they are readily available when I get the urge for a snack or want to add fresh veggies to a meal.

My kitchen is in the center of my home and is the perfect spot to place a big bowl of fresh fruit on the center island. I work from home, so I often walk by the kitchen, and each time I do, I grab a piece of fruit. A handful of grapes or blueberries is a perfect snack; placing these items in plain view reminds me to eat fruit throughout the day. The best part is I eat my fruit without thinking about it.

We are all guilty of mindlessly dipping our hands into the chip bowl until the bowl is empty. Why not replace it with fruit? As I am writing this book, it is mango season. A big bowl of delicious mango sits on my counter, saying, "Eat me." Bananas are a counter staple near the stove top where I make oatmeal. If I see it, I will eat it.

You don't have to stop with your kitchen counter. Create multiple spaces that invite you to reach for healthy foods. We stop to look at pretty things, so make your food pretty. Place cut-up fruit and veggies in clear containers so that you can see them. Place nuts and seeds in glass mason jars to remind you to add them to salads and oatmeal. When you open the refrigerator, you will see all these pretty foods on display. Make the healthy foods so visually appealing that you can't help but eat them.

This tip is simple and realistic, and best of all, it is a great way to get the kiddos to grab healthy foods, too. You may have seen advertisements for refrigerators with glass doors. The food inside looks so good you want to jump into the ad and steal the strawberries. Guess what? You don't need a fancy clear refrigerator door to have pretty fruit. You only need fresh fruit and clear containers to create the visual effect.

Create a visually appealing space anywhere you store food. Pantries are cluttered with snacks, half-eaten boxes of cereal, and pasta boxes. Start by throwing away the old, stale food and start fresh with healthy snack items, a variety of whole grains, and beans. Place the healthy options in clear containers that will entice you to grab them for an afternoon pick-me-up or when you are unsure what to make for dinner.

An organized and visually pleasing pantry is the starting point for creating delicious and nutritious meals. Your new environment will motivate you to prepare a healthy dinner with the foods that you have beautifully on display. In my house, my husband calls this "pick and pull." This is when we have no idea what to make for dinner, so we pick and pull ingredients from the pantry and refrigerator to create an amazing dinner. Get inspired! It all starts by creating an attractive space that motivates you and reinforces healthy eating. You can do this for your workspace, too.

This tip is fun, visually attractive, and helps to prevent food waste. I can't wait for you to get started today.

Summary:

- When you see or smell food, Ghrelin is released into the bloodstream, resulting in a spike in your appetite and the trigger to eat.

- Foods that are in plain view are more likely to be consumed.

- If you see it, you are more likely to eat it.

- Choose see-through containers to create a visually appealing atmosphere to encourage you to eat healthy foods.

- An organized and visually pleasing pantry is the starting point for creating delicious and nutritious meals.

Achievable Actions:

- Place fruit and vegetables in plain view so that you see them. This can be at your desk at work, kitchen counter, refrigerator, or pantry.

- Declutter your refrigerator and pantry by discarding old food and unhealthy options.

- Store healthy foods in clear containers to create a visually appealing atmosphere inviting you to reach for these foods as a snack or ingredients for your next meal.

Day 14

Go to Bed

As children, our parents made us go to bed early. They knew a good night's rest was necessary to avoid grumpy kiddos in the morning and create good little studious pupils during the day. They also made us eat breakfast. We had a nighttime and morning routine which our body became accustomed to. Until summer break came rolling around. During the summer months, moms and dads were more lenient, and routines flew out the window. I don't know about you, but I always struggled the first few weeks when school resumed; getting back into the swing of things was so hard.

It seems that most adults today are on an endless summer break without a solid routine. We seem to ebb and flow with the times and whatever is streaming on TV. At what point did we stop listening to Mom and Dad and determine that staying up late and running on little sleep is an effective strategy in life? But yet, here we are. A bunch of sleep-deprived adults running around on fumes with expectations that we can be productive, creative, and motivated on only four to five hours of sleep, just like the first day of school when we were kids. Today, we are going old school, and your task is to *go to bed*.

Can't you just hear your mom's voice saying, "Time for bed"? Good. Listen to your mother and get the rest your body needs. Oh, and breakfast in the morning won't hurt you, either.

Sleep is one of the three pillars of health, in conjunction with nutrition and movement. Sleep is a fundamental part of your overall health and well-being. Sleep affects all aspects of your health and body systems, including cardiovascular, muscular, nervous, endocrine, skeletal, lymphatic, respiratory, digestive, urinary, and reproductive systems. Sleep also affects metabolism and is closely linked to weight gain and loss. Yep, you read that right. Sleep may be the best prescription if you are struggling to lose weight.

Sleep is affected by several factors and is closely related to your mind-body health and physical environment. You will spend about one-third of your life sleeping, not because you want to, but because you *need* to. The exact amount of sleep needed depends on age, with children needing more sleep than adults to support growth and development. The Centers for Disease Control and Prevention suggest that adults aged 18-64 get 7-9 hours of sleep daily. Unfortunately, the average person gets under seven hours of sleep every night, with 70 million American adults reporting chronic sleep disturbances.

For adults, getting less than seven hours of sleep per night on a regular basis has been linked with poor health outcomes, including weight gain, diabetes, high blood pressure, heart disease, stroke, and depression. On the flip side, getting sufficient sleep will:

- Enhance your immune system
- Help prevent weight gain
- Strengthen your heart
- Improve your mood
- Increase productivity and creativity
- Enhance exercise performance

- Boost your memory

When I see new clients, one of the first things I ask about is their normal sleep patterns because sleep is vital to health and weight maintenance. My personalized nutrition plans almost always include strategies to improve sleep hygiene. Sleep hygiene encompasses your environment and habits to pave the way for higher-quality sleep and overall health.

Symptoms of poor sleep hygiene include struggling to fall asleep or stay asleep, experiencing frequent sleep disturbances throughout the night, and waking up tired. A lack of consistency in sleep quantity or quality can also be a symptom of poor sleep hygiene. If you experience any of these symptoms, you are not alone. Approximately 1 in 3 adults do not regularly get the recommended amount of uninterrupted sleep they need, which may contribute to health issues such as weight gain, diabetes, and heart disease.

Getting back to sleep and weight loss, I want to clarify that sleeping eight hours a night will not result in weight loss by itself, but it can help your body from packing on the pounds. A lack of sleep affects hormonal balance. If you don't get enough sleep, your body produces ghrelin, a hormone that boosts appetite. Your body also decreases the production of leptin, a hormone that tells you when you are full and need to burn calories. Disruption of these hormones results in late-night snacking, my friend. Plus, when you don't sleep enough, you get more stressed, affecting your sleep even more. In addition, sleep deprivation causes you to crave salty, sweet foods. The same ones that you hopefully chucked from your pantry yesterday.

Who has the energy to fight off junk food cravings when you are tired? It is exhausting just thinking about it. A lack of sleep doesn't just mess with your metabolic hormones; it also affects cortisol, a stress hormone that triggers your heart to work harder.

Many of us watch TV at night and love to binge-watch the latest new series on Netflix. Although you may think it's a good idea to binge your favorite show all night, putting off a good night's rest could affect your productivity the next day. Sleep has been shown to improve concentration and promote higher cognitive function, which can help you succeed in life! But just one restless night can negatively impact your day, making it more likely that you'll make mistakes and hit an afternoon slump that a pot of coffee won't be able to fix.

Sleep increases cognitive performance and productivity and improves hand-eye coordination, reaction time, and muscle recovery, all of which are vital for physical performance. Depriving yourself of sleep can affect your responses, strength, and power. We discussed earlier in the book that exercise improves sleep. Well, sleep also improves exercise. You need both to perform at your best.

A lack of sleep can impair the ability to think clearly, form memories, learn new things, and function optimally. Sleep is necessary so the brain can grow, reorganize, restructure, and make new neural connections that allow cells to communicate. As a result, a good night's sleep can lead to better problem-solving and decision-making skills. On Day 11, we discussed strategies to overcome challenges. To tackle this task, you must be able to problem-solve. You are more likely to make unhealthy choices in the moment when you are tired.

After only one week of getting five hours of sleep or less each night, your ability to think quickly is impacted. Sleep-deprived individuals perform poorly in activities that require quick responses and attention to multiple tasks, such as driving. In addition, too little sleep puts a person at higher risk of making poor decisions because they only have the ability to focus on a desired outcome and not the consequences.

Stimulants such as caffeine or certain medications can keep you up at night. The more tired you feel, the more likely it is that you will reach for your favorite caffeinated beverage, such as coffee. And while an afternoon pick-me-up may seem a good idea, the extra caffeine late in the day could set you up for another sleepless night.

Distractions such as electronics, especially the light from the TV, cell phones, tablets, and any other electrical device, can prevent you from falling asleep. Blue wavelengths from electronic devices are beneficial during daylight hours because they boost attention, reaction times, and mood. Unfortunately, they seem to be the most disruptive at night. In addition, exposure to light at night suppresses the secretion of melatonin, a hormone that influences circadian rhythms. One of the main contributing factors to sleep disruption is those pesky lights that we have become accustomed to having on when we go to bed.

Need some help counting sheep? Create a nighttime routine to get your mind and body relaxed. Here are some tips to help you prepare for your next 7-9 hours of blissful rest:

- **Create a routine.** Go to bed and wake up at the same time every day, even on weekends, to establish a regular sleep rhythm. Just like when we were kids. And, routines don't have to be isolated to a bedtime routine. You can also create a routine in the evening to relax. For example, grab a book and a cup of mint tea after dinner to help with digestion and quiet the mind after a long day.

- **Be mindful.** Before bedtime, try a relaxation strategy incorporating mindfulness, deep breathing, or meditation. You can do this on your own or through an app. Individuals who engage in nighttime mindfulness experience less anxiety, stress, depression, and daytime fatigue.

- **Shut it down.** The blue light emitted by digital devices such as TVs, phones, laptops, and tablets can throw off your body's internal clock. It is best to avoid them before bedtime by finding a tech-free way to wind down. You can minimize light in your sleep space by using blackout curtains or a sleep mask.

- **Don't binge-watch.** Avoid binge-watching your favorite shows at night. This will stimulate your mind and make it challenging to sleep. Give yourself at least 30 minutes to wind down and take advantage of whatever makes you feel calm and relaxed, such as soft music, light stretching, reading, and relaxation exercises.

- **Take a hot bath or shower to relax.** Going from warm water into a cooler bedroom will cause your body temperature to drop, naturally making you feel sleepy and ready to rest.

- **Enjoy essential oils.** Research demonstrates that smell affects sleep. Incorporating certain essential oils into your nightly routine can help to promote better sleep. Opt for lavender, rose, chamomile, Ylang-Ylang, peppermint, and bergamot for a restful sleep.

- **Count sheep.** I know, I know. It might sound a little silly, but it works. Allowing your brain to focus helps you power down.

- **Deep breathing.** If counting sheep isn't your thing, try focusing on your breathing by consciously taking deep breaths in and out. You can also focus on a mantra by repeating a phrase over and over. For example, repeat the words "My mind is calm and still" until you drift off to deep sleep. Other mantras you can try are:

- I welcome sleep
- I choose to sleep
- Relax, release, rest
- I deserve to rest
- Let it go

- **Create an environment that promotes rest.** The optimal sleep temperature is between 60-72 degrees Fahrenheit. Turn down your thermostat before bed or open a window on a cool night. You can also try cooling pillows and bedding.

- **Watch your intake.** Avoid caffeine, alcohol, large meals, and drinking a lot of fluid for several hours before bedtime. If you use nicotine, avoid nicotine-based substances four hours before bedtime. Nicotine has stimulant properties that are associated with sleep disruptions.

- **Exercise Regularly.** Exercise is a great stress reliever and has been shown to improve sleep quality. Do more intense workouts earlier in the day, as these will likely keep you up at night. Try to get your workouts in at least three hours before bedtime.

- **De-stress.** Sleeping is nearly impossible when you have thoughts racing through your head. Plan for 15 minutes during the day to process these thoughts. Writing a to-do list for tomorrow or brainstorming solutions can be a healthy way to deal with stress and prevent it from interfering with sleep.

- **Herbal tea.** Chamomile and other herbal teas can help relax the mind and are soothing. Try pairing it with a good book and making it part of your bedtime routine.

- **Get out of bed.** If you are having trouble falling asleep, get out of bed and do a quiet, relaxing screen-free activity; only return to bed when you can't resist falling asleep. Give that cup of tea and book a try.

- **Manage nighttime noise.** Earplugs, noise-canceling headphones, a loud fan, or a noise machine can block out disruptive nighttime sounds.

- **Limit daytime naps.** Long daytime naps can interfere with nighttime sleep. Limit naps to no more than one hour and avoid napping late in the day.

- **Contact your health provider.** Everyone has an occasional sleepless night. However, if you often have trouble sleeping or staying asleep, contact your healthcare provider. Identifying and treating any underlying causes can help you get your desired sleep.

The best way to incorporate these tips and boost your sleep hygiene is to set a sleep schedule, follow a nightly routine, and cultivate healthy habits daily. For example:

Create a sleep schedule:

- Go to bed and wake up at the same time each day
- Prioritize sleep
- Limit naps

Follow a nighttime routine:

- Get ready for bed (brush your teeth, take a shower, put on comfy PJs)
- Dim the lights
- Disconnect from electronics 30-60 minutes before bed
- Relax (meditation, reading, deep breathing, listen to soft music, or light stretches)
- Don't toss and turn (get up and read, or any calm, device-free activity, if you can't fall asleep after 20 minutes)
- Aromatherapy

Cultivate healthy habits daily:

- Be physically active
- Hydrate
- Get daylight exposure, especially sunlight, as this helps establish a healthy circadian rhythm
- Limit alcohol intake
- Avoid caffeine in the afternoon and evening
- Don't go to bed on a full stomach

Oh, and stop looking at your phone. Those social media alerts and emails will all be there in the morning. Sweet dreams!

Summary:

- Sleep is one of the three pillars of health in conjunction with nutrition and movement.

- You will spend about one-third of your life sleeping, not because you want to, but because it is essential.

- Not only does sleep increase cognitive performance and productivity, but it also improves hand-eye coordination, reaction time, and muscle recovery.

- Exposure to light suppresses the secretion of melatonin, a hormone that influences circadian rhythms.

- Researchers have linked short sleep to increased risk for depression, as well as diabetes and cardiovascular disease.

Achievable Actions:

- Establish good sleep hygiene by creating a sleep schedule and nighttime routine and cultivating healthy daily habits.

- Schedule downtime at least 30-60 minutes before bedtime to unwind, disconnect from electronics, and relax before bed. I have provided a list of tips; today, try at least 2-3 strategies tonight to promote more restful sleep.

- Download my sleep diary at www.tammyfogarty.com to monitor your sleep hygiene.

Day 15

Hey, Your Gut Is Leaking

When was the last time someone asked, "How's your gut feeling?"

Outside of your annual physical, there is likely minimal conversation about gut health between you and your doctor. If your gut is healthy, chances are, you are in good health. But an unhealthy gut can lead to a handful of issues, such as skin irritation, food sensitivities, seasonal allergies, brain fog, hormonal imbalances, digestive issues, and mood swings. Okay, so it can lead to more than a handful of issues, which is why I am compelled to discuss gut health with you today.

Gut health is a complex topic I love to discuss because most people don't realize there is a colony of bacteria residing in your gut, waiting to be fed. What you feed that colony can affect many aspects of your life, such as your mood, immune system, and how you manage stress. This colony is known as your microflora, which plays a role in gut health, inflammation, and mental health.

The gut refers to your gastrointestinal (GI) system, also known as the digestive system, and the health of your gut is generally determined by the colony of bacteria residing in your GI tract. The GI tract includes the mouth, esophagus, stomach, small intestine, large intestine, rectum, and anus. To understand the impact of gut health, it's important to understand how the gut works.

During digestion, nutrients are absorbed through the intestinal lining and transported to the bloodstream. Think of the intestinal lining as a wall that acts as a barrier between your gut and bloodstream, allowing nutrients to be delivered to different parts of your body and preventing potentially harmful substances from entering the body. When functioning properly, the intestinal lining forms a tight barrier, called junctions, to control what gets absorbed into the bloodstream.

Within our GI tract is a host of important bacteria that strengthen the intestinal lining and support the immune system. Good digestive health results from a balance of good and bad bacteria. The gut uses nerves, bacteria, and hormones to regulate digestion and to allow the brain and GI tract to communicate effectively. Cross-talk between the brain and gut could be along the lines of "It's time to eat; let's release digestive enzymes to prepare for digestion" or "Hey, this body has had enough to eat; let's send the signal we're full." While the gut and brain communicate, we must listen to the cues our body sends us to determine whether we are hungry, satisfied, ate too much, and most importantly, feel bloated, in pain, or have food intolerances, all of which may be a sign of GI inflammation, or possibly leaky gut.

Listening to your gut is about more than responding to your body when you get that "gut feeling" or need to make a decision. Your gut health can substantially affect your mood, immune system, and more. Here are some signs that your body may be telling you something is not right in your gut:

- Poor gut health is associated with minor but unpleasant effects on the body, such as abdominal pain, bloating, acid reflux, and flatulence.
- Headaches, chronic fatigue, and joint pain may indicate a leaky gut.
- Brain fog and difficulty concentrating can be related to the health of your microflora.
- Mood imbalances, including depression and anxiety, can also indicate a leaky gut.

As I mentioned, the intestinal lining acts as a barrier between your gut and bloodstream to prevent potentially harmful substances from entering your body. An unhealthy gut may weaken the walls of the GI tract, resulting in cracks or holes. These cracks or holes are actually the weakening of the junctions that hold the wall together tightly. Weak junctions allow partially digested food, toxins, and bacteria to enter the bloodstream, known as leaky gut syndrome.

Leaky gut syndrome, defined by the medical community as "increased intestinal permeability," may let toxins into your bloodstream triggering an inflammatory response. Over time, chronic inflammation can manifest in various diseases, such as inflammatory bowel disease, celiac disease, autoimmune disorders, depression, anxiety, arthritis, fibromyalgia, obesity, diabetes, asthma, and chronic fatigue.

While leaky gut is not currently a recognized medical diagnosis, the theory explains various conditions that medical doctors haven't been able to fully explain yet. We know that the condition of having intestinal permeability, or a "leaky gut," is real, but the verdict is still out there if it is an actual disease or if a leaky gut causes other diseases.

Right now, we understand the symptoms associated with a leaky gut, and the good news is that there is a way to repair and strengthen the walls of your GI tract so you don't spring any "leaks."

Your choices may actually be the main driver of gut inflammation. Research shows that the standard American diet (aka: SAD), which is low in fiber and high in sugar and saturated fats, may initiate this process. Heavy alcohol use and stress also seem to disrupt this microflora balance, contributing to inflammation.

Since leaky gut syndrome isn't an official diagnosis, no medical treatment is recommended. But you can do plenty of things to improve your overall digestive health and improve symptoms associated with GI inflammation and leaky gut. One is to eat a diet rich in foods that aid the growth of healthy bacteria.

Before I provide a list of choices to improve your gut health, it is important to notice just how expansive the colony of bacteria inside you really is. There are anywhere from 50-100 trillion bacteria in your body. Yes, TRILLION. Most bacteria reside in your gut, known as the gut microbiome.

Hundreds of species of bacteria are in your intestines, each of which plays a specific role in health and requires different nutrients for growth. The more diverse your diet is with grains, beans, and a variety of fruits and vegetables, the more diverse your microbiome will be, contributing to overall health and wellness. Unfortunately, the SAD diet is not very diverse; thus, most people walk around with gut colonies overrun by bacteria that may do more harm than good. The good news is that you can shake up your colony by adding foods that promote a balanced variety of microflora. Let's start with prebiotics and probiotics.

Probiotics are living microscopic bacteria or yeasts proven to support healthy digestive and immune systems. These "good" microbes are the same or similar beneficial bacteria found in healthy microbiomes and certain fermented foods and supplements.

Prebiotics are found in fiber-rich plant foods, including fruits, vegetables, whole grains, nuts, and legumes. These foods contain a certain type of fiber called insoluble fiber that we cannot digest. The nondigestible fiber travels to our large intestines and provides "food" for the probiotics. Prebiotics support the growth and activity of probiotics. Without prebiotics, probiotics can't thrive or reproduce. By simply eating a fiber-rich diet, we support the growth of healthy bacteria.

The difference between probiotics and prebiotics is that probiotics are live beneficial organisms, and prebiotics are the food they need to survive.

Prebiotics

- **Vegetables:** broccoli, arugula, carrots, kale, spinach, zucchini, artichoke, asparagus, cabbage, chicory root, garlic, jicama, leeks, mushroom, onion, shallot, sweet potato, tomato, collard greens, dandelion greens, mustard greens, and chard

- **Fruit:** strawberries, raspberries, apples, pears, banana, blueberries, cranberry, kiwifruit, guava, passion fruit, and pomegranate

- **Grains:** barley, wheat bran, rice bran, corn, oats, rice, whole grain wheat

- **Legumes:** chickpeas, lentils, peas, soybeans, and dry beans

- **Nuts and seeds:** almonds, pistachios, cashews, walnuts, flaxseeds

Because different probiotic species prefer different prebiotic foods, it's best to eat a wide variety of foods from this list daily. *Please note: this list is an example of foods to consume and does not include all the foods that promote a healthy gut.*

Probiotics

People have consumed foods that contain probiotics for thousands of years, deeply rooted in ancient cultures, including kefir, kimchi, kombucha, miso, pickled vegetables, sauerkraut, and yogurt. For most healthy people, a probiotic supplement is unnecessary, and foods are the best source of probiotics. However, supplementation can be beneficial for certain conditions using specific species of probiotics. Since foods are my first choice, I will not discuss probiotic supplementation in the book, but you can visit www.tammyfogarty.com to read more about supplementation and determine if it is right for you.

A diet rich in fermented foods enhances the diversity of the gut microbiome. Fermentation is a process in which live cultures, such as bacteria and yeast, break down sugars. Fermented foods can enhance the gut microbiome, creating a healthy mix of microbes that strengthen the walls of the intestines.

It is important to note that not all fermented foods are created equal. Live cultures are found in yogurt and a yogurt-like drink called kefir. Fermented vegetables contain live cultures due to fermentation, including sauerkraut, pickles, and Korean pickled vegetables (kimchi). The jars of pickles you can buy from the grocery are often pickled using vinegar and not the natural fermentation process using live organisms, which means they don't contain probiotics. To ensure the fermented foods you choose contain probiotics, look for the words "naturally fermented" or "contains live active cultures" on the label.

I encourage you to add fermented foods to your diet. Start by finding tasty recipes that use the following **fermented foods**:

- Tempeh
- Natto
- Miso
- Kimchi
- Sauerkraut
- Probiotic Yogurt

Fermented beverages include:

- Kefir
- Kombucha

Foods to limit

Some foods have been shown to cause inflammation in your body, which may promote the growth of unhealthy gut bacteria that are linked to many chronic diseases. The following list contains foods that may disrupt healthy microflora as well as some that are believed to trigger digestive symptoms, such as bloating, constipation, and diarrhea:

- **Refined carbohydrates:** refined bread, pasta, cereals
- **Processed meats:** cold cuts, deli meats, bacon, hot dogs
- **Baked goods:** cookies, cakes, muffins, pies, pastries
- **Snack/junk foods:** crackers, granola bars, pretzels, chips, candy bars, ice cream
- **Refined oils:** canola, sunflower, soybean, and safflower oils
- **Artificial sweeteners:** aspartame, sucralose, and saccharin
- **Beverages:** alcohol, carbonated beverages, and other sugary drinks

While I am not suggesting that you self-diagnose yourself with leaky gut syndrome, I do want you to be aware of how foods make you feel and how you feel in general. Bloating, gas, constipation, diarrhea, abdominal pain, skin irritation, and headaches are not normal. After your physician has determined there are no health concerns, it is up to you to decide the next steps to alleviate these symptoms. Monitor how certain foods make you feel; your diet may be the culprit, causing you to feel symptoms related to GI inflammation. The good news is that you have the ability to change your diet and include foods and nutrients that reduce inflammation.

One of my favorite quotes is from Ann Wigmore, the founder of the Hippocrates Health Institute, *"The food you eat can either be the safest and most powerful form of medicine or the slowest form of poison."* Let that resonate for a moment. You have a choice today to heal your gut, reduce inflammation, and feel better simply by choosing foods that work for your body, rather than against your body.

What do you say we start working on that gut together? Which Achievable Actions will you implement today?

Summary:

- During digestion, nutrients are absorbed through the intestinal lining and transported to the bloodstream.

- The health of your gut is generally determined by the colony of bacteria residing in your GI tract.

- While leaky gut is not currently a recognized medical diagnosis, the theory explains various conditions that medical doctors haven't been able to fully explain yet.

- Hundreds of species of bacteria are in your intestines, each of which plays a specific role in health and requires different nutrients for growth.

- The more diverse your diet is with grains, beans, and a variety of fruits and vegetables, the more diverse your microbiome will be, contributing to overall health and wellness.

- The difference between probiotics and prebiotics is that probiotics are live beneficial organisms, and prebiotics are the food they need to survive.

- "The food you eat can either be the safest and most powerful form of medicine or the slowest form of poison." – Ann Wigmore

Achievable Actions:

- Include 1-2 prebiotic foods at each meal. Prebiotic foods include fruit, vegetables, grains, legumes, nuts, and seeds.

- Try a new recipe that includes fermented food such as kimchi, tempeh, or probiotic yogurt.

- Practice the Mindful Eating technique to determine how these foods make you feel.

- Visit www.tammyfogarty.com to download the Food Diary to track how you feel once you have included pre- and probiotics in your daily routine.

Day 16

You Are One Bite Away From a Good Mood

Disclaimer:

This section may contain content that explores themes related to mental health, including but not limited to depression, anxiety, and other emotional challenges. It is important to be aware that engaging with this material may evoke emotional responses. If you or someone you know is struggling with mental health issues, it is crucial to seek professional help. This book is not a substitute for mental health treatment, therapy, or counseling. Consult a qualified mental health professional for personalized guidance and support. Take care of yourself while reading this book. If any of the content is causing distress, it is okay to take a break or skip ahead. Prioritize your mental and emotional well-being.

Have you ever binge-watched your favorite reality show after a crappy day, mindlessly reaching for the last bit of broken chips at the bottom of the bag? If so, you know a little something about the relationship between food and your mood. We have high hopes that a pint of ice cream or a large cheese pizza will create a better mood. While emotional eating is real, the relationship between food and actual mood disorders, such as depression and anxiety, is not so cut and dry.

As I mentioned yesterday, gut health is a complex topic that expands beyond what I have already shared with you. One of the most fascinating aspects of gut health is how it relates to our ever-changing moods. Research has demonstrated that certain nutrients can improve concentration, increase alertness, enhance problem-solving skills, and boost productivity. We also understand the consequences of a poor diet can result in:

- Fatigue
- Decreased mental effectiveness
- Increased irritability
- Decreased energy levels
- Reduced ability to think clearly and make decisions
- Decreased job performance and productivity

On the flip side, a healthy diet is associated with:

- Sustained energy
- Improved digestion
- Increased concentration
- Enhanced productivity

I want you to take a moment to think about when you are the most productive. What environment do you thrive in? What motivates you?

"Food" is not the reply that usually comes to mind when I ask that question. But, it should be a factor to consider if you want to feel energized, productive, creative, and just to be freakin' happy. Personally, food plays a significant factor in how I perform. As I was writing this chapter, I took a break to have lunch. The process of eating lunch doesn't typically require much thought; however, I approach food with careful consideration because the foods I eat will absolutely affect how I feel and, ultimately, my mood.

Today for lunch, I opted for leftover chicken and spinach meatballs and a salad of mixed greens, with cherry tomatoes drizzled with lemon olive oil and balsamic vinegar. Had I chosen differently, I may not be sitting here writing about my lunch and, instead, would be sitting on the couch watching the next episode of *Selling Sunset* on Netflix.

My other option was sliders from yesterday's BBQ. I love a good mini burger topped with American cheese. The problem with sliders is that they are mini, and we often perceive "mini" with the notion of "I need to eat two or three because they are small." Some mini things pack a powerful punch, including mini burgers. Regardless of the size, the bread and cheese will affect my ability to concentrate, ultimately killing my mojo to continue writing this book for you today. So, chicken meatballs and salad it is!

By practicing the Mindful Eating techniques I shared with you on Day 6, as well as using the food journal from my website, you can identify how certain foods make you feel. I actively practice mindful eating, and it has changed my life because I have also been able to determine which foods make me feel more productive and creative. This combination of the right foods and my mood makes me feel good. When I feel good, I am confident. I am happy. I have a purpose. Don't you want to feel this, too? I know you do.

But I haven't always felt this way. It took me a while to figure out. Heck, I spent years running through fast-food restaurants and giving in to my pizza and pasta cravings, wondering why I always felt tired and dragging ass. I was easily distracted and struggled to keep up with my to-do list. Too often, I had to dig deep to find an ounce of motivation to get through the day.

Some days, my only motivation was a couple of glasses of wine and a big heaping plate of feel-good comfort food.

This lifestyle, despite being a dietitian, went on for years. I was great at telling people what to do, but I wasn't so great at following my own advice. I tend to take on too many tasks, and so I often burn the candle at both ends. At the time, I had no clue about gut health. I did not realize that my diet was affecting how I performed each day. As I learned about the colony residing in my gut, I better understood why I felt so down in the dumps and unmotivated to make any changes. My friend, I have a feeling that you, too, experience the same symptoms. But, you can take control of how you feel.

Can it be that easy?

Can foods make you more productive?

Can food be the driving force you have been looking for?

Can simple dietary changes improve your mood?

Yes! The answer is YES. Today, you will choose foods that improve your mood. I like to call it *Food for Your Mood.*

As you learned yesterday, the food you choose to eat directly nourishes the microflora in your gut. Feed yourself junk, and you will produce junky bacteria that can negatively impact your body. However, if your diet includes a variety of fruit, vegetables, whole grains, healthy fats, and lean protein, your microflora will flourish to promote health, restore and maintain balance, and enhance your mood. It all starts with your second brain.

It's long been known that the brain communicates with the GI tract. When you are upset or feel stressed, you feel it in your gut. This is because your brain sends signals to the digestive tract that trigger GI symptoms, such as an upset stomach. But, the communication goes both ways; hence, the gut is referred to as your "second brain." The GI tract also sends signals, and when you are dealing with an inflamed GI, it can send signals to the brain that can affect your mood or disrupt your sleep. This bi-directional communication is called the Gut-Brain Axis.

The gut-brain axis likely explains why individuals with mental health disorders, such as depression and anxiety, report GI issues such as changes in appetite, weight gain or loss, diarrhea, and nausea. Alternatively, individuals diagnosed with GI issues such as irritable bowel syndrome and inflammatory bowel disease report feeling stressed and experiencing mood disturbances, anxiety, and depression. It has to do with the cross-talk between the brain and your gut.

But wait, there's more! The term "gut microbiota-brain axis" refers to the communication between the brain and the bacteria that naturally live in the gut and the influence the gut microbes have on the brain. Hormones, nerves, and neurotransmitters all help make this communication possible.

One communication route is via the vagus nerve, which runs from the base of the brain to the digestive system. For example, the brain signals and sends instructions via the vagus nerve to the stomach to release gastric acid and digestive enzymes when food is present. In turn, the stomach does a good job communicating with the brain through the vagus nerve, so you eat when you are hungry and stop eating once you feel full.

The gut bacteria produce neurotransmitters such as serotonin, dopamine, and GABA. These neurotransmitters play a vital role in mood, depression, and anxiety. In fact, approximately 90 percent of the body's serotonin is produced in the gut and regulates cognition and mood. This hopefully gives you a whole new perspective on "that gut feeling."

Fruit and vegetables contain vital nutrients that foster the production of dopamine, a neurotransmitter that plays a role in curiosity, motivation, and engagement. Alternatively, consuming a diet with processed carbohydrates, too much protein, saturated fat, and refined sugar increases levels of tryptophan. An increase in tryptophan causes the brain to increase the production of serotonin, a neurotransmitter that helps regulate sleep. No wonder you are falling asleep at your desk! Your footlong sub is putting you to sleep.

If you want to avoid the afternoon slump and the dumpy mood that comes along with it, avoid the following foods, especially during the day:

- Processed food
- High-fat dairy
- Red meat
- Saturated fat
- Sodium
- Refined sugar
- Refined grains

Depression and anxiety are the most common mental health conditions worldwide, making them a leading cause of disability. According to the World Health Organization, depression is the fourth most common global burden of disease. What most do not realize is that you don't have to be diagnosed with depression to feel symptoms. We can all feel down in the dumps, but for some, it is more debilitating than in others.

Subclinical symptoms of mental health are low-level and short-lived mental or emotional drawbacks that can affect your personal and professional life. It is important to note that the choices you make in each moment, such as what to eat, whether to exercise, and hours of sleep, can result in subclinical symptoms of mental health affecting how you feel and contributing to your mood.

While I am not suggesting that it's possible to identify a single nutritional factor that increases or decreases the risk of depression, one can assess how foods make them feel. For example, the Mediterranean diet, which is actually a lifestyle more than a diet, is rich in fruits, vegetables, olive oil, whole grains, and lean protein such as chicken and fish and low in red meat and unhealthy fats. This dietary pattern is associated with lower blood pressure, better cognitive function, and lower incidence of diabetes and cardiovascular events. The overall healthy, high-quality dietary pattern is associated with a decreased incidence of depression and anxiety. Regular physical activity has also been shown to enhance mood and may decrease symptoms of depression and anxiety.

By making the choice to eat healthy foods, get sufficient rest, drink enough water, and exercise, you are making the choice to feel good. This lifestyle is associated with increased productivity, creativity, improved problem-solving, and overall quality of life. Who has time to feel anxious or moody when they feel this good?

You are literally one bite away from a good mood. Give it a try today. Continue to nourish your body with a variety of fruits, vegetables, whole grains, healthy fat, and lean protein. These foods will create the healthy microflora that directs the brain and gut to effectively communicate to enhance your mood. In the end, you win. You win BIG! You will feel great and be better equipped to make healthy choices continuously.

In addition, I want you to take a moment to reflect on the achievable actions that were easy for you to accomplish. I also want you to reflect on the ones that you are avoiding. We tend to avoid the things that we need the most. Everything in this book is meant to enhance your well-being and empower your ability to make healthy choices in every moment.

What are you hesitant to change?

What obstacles are in your way?

Now, take a moment to reflect and come up with a plan to do the things you don't want to do. Take the leap. It's okay to feel unsettled in the moment as long as it leads to a healthy change. Overcoming obstacles motivates you to do more. What is next on your list? If you are not sure, I have a list of Achievable Actions waiting for you below. You got this, my friend. Get on with it.

Summary:

- Research has demonstrated that certain nutrients can improve concentration, increase alertness, enhance problem-solving skills, and boost productivity.

- Feed yourself junk, and you will produce junky bacteria that can negatively impact your body.

- With a variety of fruits, vegetables, whole grains, healthy fats, and lean protein, your microflora will flourish to promote health, restore and maintain balance, and enhance your mood.

- Fruit and vegetables contain vital nutrients that foster the production of dopamine, a neurotransmitter that plays a role in curiosity, motivation, and engagement.

- Approximately 90 percent of the body's serotonin is produced in the gut and regulates cognition and mood.

Achievable Actions:

- You must consume a variety of foods to obtain a healthy balance of nutrients. The more colorful your foods, the more nutrients you get. Today, add 1-2 new healthy, colorful foods to your meals. These foods can be fruits, veggies, grains, nuts, seeds, herbal tea, etc.

- Use the Food Journal found on www.tammyfogarty.com to record how certain foods make you feel. Do they enhance your mood or negatively affect your mood?

- Try at least one achievable action that you have avoided.

Day 17

Have a Plan

My husband and I have a yearly tradition of spending our anniversary skiing. On one trip, I expressed how much fun it would be to go sledding. After three years of sharing my desire to go sledding, Rob finally agreed, and it was a day I will never forget.

Dressed in our ski pants and jackets, we got a two-person sled from the hotel's front desk, along with a strict warning not to get caught and to stay away from the ski lift. I was beyond excited and felt like a little kid. It was late at night, and no one was around; we were going to have so much fun!

Rob settled into the back of the sled while I climbed in front, and off we went. Unfortunately, we only made it about two feet because my feet dragged and slowed us down. Laughing at my mistake, I rearranged my position on the sled and prepared for the next attempt. One, two, three... here we go! Whoa. That was not what I expected.

Before I could process what just happened, we were covered from head to toe in snow at the bottom of the hill. It is a good thing my husband aborted mission because we steered off course and would have crashed into the ski lift. Much to my dismay, sledding was not as fun as I expected. I loved it and hated it at the same time.

Had we planned better, we could have dominated that slope. The ski pants were smart, but we didn't consider a helmet to protect our heads if we ran into something or goggles to shield our eyes from the freezing snow barreling into our faces. Oh, and gloves. Gloves would have been a great idea. I was determined to get it right next year.

The following year, we decided to give sledding another try and chose the last night of the trip to conquer the slope. This time, we were ready. Ski pants, jackets, goggles, ski gloves, and, most importantly, helmets. We had everything we needed. Except for a sled.

The point of the story is that a goal without a plan creates disappointment. The same can be said for your lifestyle choices. If you don't plan to eat healthy, exercise, or prepare for rest, you will face unintended consequences and disappointment. I assumed the sled would be there, waiting for us. My sledding adventures will have to wait until next year. But today, I can plan for other important events, such as ensuring I always have healthy foods on hand.

I plan my day. Every day. From what I will eat, when to work out, and which tasks to complete. I haven't always been a planner, but as I get older and wiser, I realize that if I don't plan my day, I walk around aimlessly, multitasking and ending my day saying, "Crap, I forgot to do that."

One of the most important plans is what I eat during the week. And it extends beyond what foods I will put in my mouth. I plan to get the most meals from my available foods. My time is precious, and as much as I love cooking, I hate doing dishes and don't want to spend too much time cooking and cleaning up the huge mess I always make. I aim to cook only a few meals but have enough food to prepare several. It's a simple strategy. It's as simple as sledding down a hill as long as you have a plan.

The first step is to pick a recipe. I determine what I can do with the leftover ingredients to prepare other meals from that one recipe. In addition, my lunches throughout the week largely come from leftover dinners. You need to start here:

- Plan for at least three dinners.
- Choose meal options that have similar ingredients so you have less food waste.
- Make extra that can be used for tomorrow's dinner.
- Your leftovers make the perfect lunch.

My three main meals/recipes:

1. Grilled Whole Chicken
2. Shephard's Pie
3. Grilled Steak

Day 1 Dinner: Grilled whole chicken with mashed potatoes, salad, and roasted carrots.

- Make extra mashed potatoes and carrots to be used for tomorrow's shepherd's pie recipe.
- Make a huge salad. Tomorrow's lunch will be a grilled chicken salad.
  - *Tip: Don't add the dressing since it will wilt your veggies.*

Day 2 Lunch: Salad with grilled chicken.

- Lunch will consist of salad from last night's dinner and chicken diced into bite-sized pieces.

Day 2 Dinner: Ground turkey shepherd's pie with a side salad.

Day 3 Lunch: Leftover shepherd's pie, because it tastes better the next day.

Day 3 Dinner: Grilled steak with roasted sweet potato and Mediterranean quinoa.

- Make an extra sweet potato and quinoa so that you can prepare lunch for the next day.
- Make extra steak for dinner and lunch later in the week.

Day 4 Lunch: Black bean and sweet potato quinoa bowl.

- The extra sweet potato and Mediterranean quinoa you made yesterday is today's lunch.

Day 4 Dinner: Salad with grilled steak.

- If you make a big enough salad on Monday, you may have salad for today. I always make a HUGE salad that lasts throughout the week. The key is to avoid ingredients that will wilt the greens.

Day 5 Lunch: Mediterranean quinoa with grilled steak.

Day 5 Dinner: It's Friday! Treat yourself and have a night out. Check out Day 20 for healthy tips for dining out.

As you can see, you can have food available for the entire week by just preparing a few meals and side dishes. The goal is to prepare large portions while you are in the kitchen so that you can use the remaining food to create lunch or dinner the next day. My husband likes to call this the "pick and pull" method. We pull out leftover food and pick ingredients on hand to create delicious meals without spending too much time in the kitchen.

Not a fan of leftovers? Change your mindset. Don't think of it as leftover food. Why not make it easy on yourself by making extra food to prepare effortless meals later in the week? Most importantly, you will have healthy foods available to make healthy choices in the moment. Lastly, plan meals that share ingredients to eliminate extra food waste. Choose recipes that call for the same veggies, protein, and herbs.

My version of meal planning means I don't have to think about what I will eat for lunch or ponder what's for dinner after a long day. When you fail to plan your meals, you will find yourself ordering a pizza or running through the drive-thru. Don't get stuck without healthy options. You have a choice to fill your refrigerator with foods that will nourish your body, and you have a choice to make extra food so that you are not cooking every day. Here is another example of how you can plan your week:

Day 1 Dinner: Ground turkey and spicy Italian sausage empanadas with a side salad.

- I love empanadas. They are easy to make and kid-friendly. Empanadas are filled with protein, such as ground beef or shredded chicken. Whatever protein you use, make extra to have tacos for dinner the next night.

- Reserve 2 hot Italian sausage links and some ground turkey to make chili later in the week.

- Make a BIG salad to add to your meals throughout the week.

Day 2 Lunch: Empanadas and a salad.

Day 2 Dinner: Turkey chili with spicy (or sweet) Italian sausage and cornbread muffins with a side salad.

Day 3 Lunch: A bowl of chili and cornbread because this is even better than shepherd's pie the next day. Or a cup of chili and an empanada.

Day 3 Dinner: Tacos! Use the remaining empanada filling to make tacos. Use leftover ingredients from your salad, such as diced radishes, green onions, and cilantro as taco toppings.

Day 4 Lunch: Tacos and a side salad.

Day 4 Dinner: Grilled salmon, farro salad, grilled asparagus, and mixed greens

Day 5 Lunch: Farro salad with chilled asparagus.

Day 5 Dinner: Salmon cakes over mixed greens.

Life is complicated. Your meals do not have to be. Have fun with them and be creative. If cooking is not your thing or you don't have time, I suggest meal delivery programs. There are a variety of meal delivery programs that will prepare nutritious meals and have them delivered right to your door.

Another suggestion is to purchase pre-made foods from the market. I love markets with a huge display of already-cooked foods such as steak, chicken, fish, and various sides. This option will cost more money, but for some, the convenience of having someone else cook is worth it.

My final suggestion is to take cooking lessons. Cooking classes are a lot of fun and a great family activity. You will be introduced to new foods, techniques, and flavors. Have fun with cooking and explore new ideas. In addition, preparing your meals is healthier than eating at a restaurant. We don't know what is added to the foods we order, but you will know exactly what ingredients you add to your foods.

Today, I want you to choose at least three recipes with similar ingredients. Plan how you will prepare several meals for the week. Here are some tips as you plan your week:

- There are several food blogs and cooking apps available. Find one that you love. I enjoy using Pinterest or the Food Network app on my phone to find new recipes.

- Use social media for recipe ideas and cooking tips. Ina Garten is my go-to for easy recipes with fresh ingredients.

- Keep it simple! Don't choose recipes that have forty ingredients or require mad culinary skills.

- Make a BIG salad that you can add to any meal.

- Double or triple your recipes so you have extra for the next meal.

- Use fresh ingredients. Fresh ingredients will maintain their freshness throughout the week.

- Experiment with fresh and dried herbs. They can turn a bland meal into a flavor bomb.

- Choose recipes that share similar ingredients so you have less waste.

- Don't be afraid to try new things.

- Let the kiddos choose a recipe and have them help prepare meals.

Once you have your recipes, prepare a shopping list and head to the grocery store. Follow me on social media @nutritiontammy for fun recipes and ideas to get you through the week. Bon appetit!

Summary:

- A goal without a plan creates disappointment.
- Plan what you will eat during the week.
- Not a fan of leftovers? Then change your mindset.
- Don't get stuck without healthy options.
- Life is complicated. Your meals do not have to be.

Achievable Actions:

- Choose three recipes for the week.
- Make extra so you have food on hand for the next few meals.
- Make the most of your ingredients by incorporating leftover veggies, herbs, and sides into the next meal.

Day 18

Don't Break the Bank

The rising price of groceries and eating out can be a huge burden on the monthly budget. From household staples such as bread, eggs, and milk to canned goods, cleaning supplies, and body wash, it's easier than ever to break the bank at the grocery store if you're not careful. Despite the jaw-dropping prices, all hope is not lost if you shop with a plan. With the right budget-friendly tips and planning techniques, you can save money at the grocery store and cut down on food waste while you're at it.

The idea of spending less on food sounds good in theory. However, budgeting tips require you to make fundamental changes to how you behave. Yes, you read that right. We need to change our behaviors to change how we spend. Even if it feels like these changes are doable, the truth is that you spend the way you spend for a reason. Asking someone to change how they spend their hard-earned money can feel overwhelming, and you may get discouraged. So today, the focus is not on changing how you approach food spending but on transforming your current habits to reduce costs. You'll be surprised to see how much you can save by making only a few little tweaks.

Tips to save money at the grocery store:

- **Plan ahead.** Plan your meals for the week so you buy only what you need.

- **Live by the list.** Create a shopping list of ingredients needed, and don't deviate from the plan when you get to the store. I am a sucker for BOGO deals and often buy items I don't need because I can't resist a good buy-one-get-one-free deal. Not every sale is a good buy.

- **Check before you buy.** Check your pantry and refrigerator before buying new items. Duplicate items in your pantry can kill your grocery budget and quickly lead to food waste. This is how I ended up with three jars of pickles in my pantry. Use what you already have.

- **Take advantage of shopping apps.** Many grocery stores offer apps to carefully plan your shopping trip from the comfort of your own home. Don't forget to check available coupons, too. Utilizing your grocery store's app is one of the best ways to stay on budget and save time when you shop. Instacart is currently my go-to shopping app and includes fifty-two stores to shop from! I can order exactly what I need, from groceries to pet supplies to home improvement supplies, and avoid frivolous spending.

- **Opt for curbside pickup.** If the bakery and potato chip aisles are too tempting, shop ahead on your store's website or mobile app. Many stores let you choose between curbside pick-up or having it delivered. You may find curbside pickup to be more cost-effective since delivery fees can be expensive.

- **Add it up.** As you add items to your cart in the app, you can see your working total, which is super helpful when you have a set budget in mind.

- **Shop alone.** Impulse buying can be one of the costliest habits at the grocery store. Shopping with the kiddos or a partner may increase your likelihood of buying something you don't need. Rather than bringing your family members with you to the grocery store, add their requested items to your shopping list and leave the kiddos at home.

- **Avoid the hustle and bustle.** Certain times of the day are more busy, so find a quiet time to shop and avoid the crowds. Crowds can negatively impact your grocery budget because the people and noise around you can be a distraction from making cost-effective decisions.

- **Shop the perimeter.** The aisles in the center of the grocery store contain processed foods, which tend to be pricey, and not the healthiest choices. However, the perimeter is where you'll find healthy foods like fruits, vegetables, and other unprocessed foods that are more cost-effective.

- **Eye level is buy level.** Since products at eye level are most likely to get your attention, retailers often place more expensive items on these shelves. Browse all the shelves to get the most bang for your buck.

- **Buy in bulk.** Some foods are significantly cheaper when purchased in bulk. So, when it makes sense, buy in large quantities. I like purchasing meats in bulk and freezing individual portions when needed. If buying in bulk is too much for your household, ask a friend or family member if they want to split the purchase with you.

- **Don't shop when you're hungry.** This tip is an oldy but a goody. Going to a grocery store when you're hungry results in grabbing groceries you don't need. Instead, eat a meal or snack before heading to the store so you're not focused on your hunger pangs.

- **Purchase in-season produce.** Out-of-season produce tends to be more expensive than its in-season counterparts. Determine what is in season and choose recipes that include those items. Frozen produce is also a great alternative to fresh; you can purchase it year-round, and it's usually less expensive.

- **Use what you buy.** We all get excited to try a new recipe to get motivated to cook for an army. This is great, but use what you buy. Go home and prep those meals while you are excited and motivated. Otherwise, you will have wasted money while the abundance of produce is rotting away in the refrigerator.

The Cost of Convenience

Suppose you had two $1 bills. You take one, spend it on something useful, and throw the other $1 down the garbage disposal. You may feel a little bad, but it's just a dollar. What's a dollar in the grand scheme of things? But what if you had two $50 bills? You spend one and light the second $50 with a match to watch it burn. For most of us, watching that $50 bill go up in flames will hurt. Wasting larger amounts of money becomes harder to ignore. So what if I told you that you are currently wasting a lot of money regularly?

We are all guilty of wasting food... and a lot of money! Do you buy food you don't use (I am totally guilty of this), make too much food, and throw away the leftovers? Do you utilize all the ingredients on hand? Have you ever found a food item while rummaging through your pantry and asked, "Where did you come from?" If you answer yes to any of these questions, then you are wasting money, my friend. If you want to save money, you have to stop wasting money.

The key to avoiding wasting food and money is to be mindful of what you already have. The things you have in the refrigerator or pantry should be first and foremost in your mind when planning your meals for the week, creating the shopping list, and before you even consider eating out.

Do you remember as a kid asking your mom or dad if you could stop at McDonald's because you're *starving*, and they would say, "We have plenty of food at home"? They said this for a reason! Because there is always plenty of food at home. When and why have we become a nation of food-wasters? Listen to your parents. Not only do we need to go to bed, we need to stop wasting food and put this bad habit to rest.

If you could save $100- $200 a month just by paying a little bit more attention to what you already have, why wouldn't you? Based on the USDA, the average family of four will spend the following on groceries each month:

- **Low-cost budget.** For a low-cost budget for a family of four, you can plan on spending $241.70 a week or about $1,047.10 a month.

- **Moderate-cost budget.** For a family of four with a moderate budget, you would spend $301.20 a week for groceries or $1,304.70 a month.

- **Liberal budget.** For a liberal budget for a family of four, you can plan on paying $363.70 a week or $1,910.60 a month.

One way to avoid wasting money is to have a Pantry Day 2-4 times per month. Pantry Day is when you only utilize what you have available in your refrigerator or pantry. As I mentioned earlier, we call this the "Pick and Pull" method in our home. There are some great apps that will provide recipes based on the ingredients you have on hand, such as Super Cook, Allrecipes, Epicurious, and Magic Fridge.

Our actions are a result of a habit. Wasting food is essentially a bad habit. It's a bad habit to buy more food than you need. It's a bad habit to buy food on sale and stash it until it expires. It's a very bad habit to buy fresh produce to watch it rot (yet again, I am guilty of this). Lastly, it's a bad habit to throw away leftovers because you "don't like leftovers." Which makes no sense because you ate that same food the day before. Don't waste it!

Habits develop through repetition and positive feedback. We can easily create new habits by breaking bad ones and replacing them with something rewarding, such as more money in your bank account. Keep in mind that you created your bad habits. You are very capable of training yourself to change your habits.

Another way to save money is to take a hard look at the cost of convenience. I love convenience, but it comes at a cost. That's not necessarily bad because some things are worth paying for. Buying groceries at a store is convenient. Having a washing machine, dishwasher, and smartphone is super convenient and worth the cost. We pay for conveniences each day.

But we need to consider the cost of conveniences that don't necessarily justify their costs, especially regarding groceries. For example, a large bag of chips will cost about 21 cents per ounce, but buying the convenient snack-size bags to throw in the kids' lunch box is 38 cents per ounce. Baby carrots are great for snacking but will cost you 8 cents per ounce as compared to 4 cents per ounce of regular carrots. Did you know that baby carrots are not actually "baby"? They are made from smaller, broken large carrots. So, you are paying more for the same things. You can get double the carrots if you peel and cut your own "baby" carrots.

Pre-sliced fruit comes with a hefty price increase. Sliced apples are approximately 33 cents per ounce compared to buying a bag of apples to peel and slice yourself at 10 cents per ounce. You will pay a premium for chicken breasts, pre-formed hamburger patties, and cauliflower rice. Instead, buy the whole chicken, make your hamburger patties, and use a food processor to cut cauliflower into rice-sized pieces.

At the end of the day, you'll still be buying the foods you love and always bought, but just a slightly less convenient version of those foods. You can handle it! Once you've grown accustomed to doing things yourself, all those conveniently packaged foods will seem less and less convenient and more like a waste of your precious money.

Summary:

- The rising price of groceries and eating out can greatly burden the monthly budget.
- With the right budget-friendly tips and planning techniques, you can save money at the grocery store and cut down on food waste while you're at it.
- You'll be surprised to see how much you can save by making only a few little tweaks.
- Habits develop through repetition and positive feedback.
- Consider the cost of conveniences that don't necessarily justify their costs, especially regarding our groceries.

Achievable Actions:

- Start slowly by choosing at least two tips to save money at the grocery store today.

- Determine which foods you pay a premium for because they are convenient. Then, I want you to try to do without that item and instead do it yourself. For example, stop buying sliced apples and slice your own, stop buying frozen cauliflower rice, and instead buy a head of cauliflower and put it into a food processor to make your cauliflower rice.

- Try your very own Pantry Day with the ingredients you have available. Use one of the apps I shared with you.

Day 19

Winning the Battle Against Overindulgence

You know that feeling when you eat something so good you don't want to stop? Food that is bursting-at-the-seams-good, causing you to unbutton your pants and get horizontal on the couch as soon as possible. Good times!

But, unfortunately, overindulging can quickly turn into a night of regret. You question your judgment, and that extra helping, as your stomach aches. The belly bloat is no joke, and you are so uncomfortable you can't wait to get home and slip into your favorite stretchy pants, all the while hoping that no one is behind you as you pass gas. Been there. Done that. But why go back there?

Certain foods make me weak, like pasta and tacos. I love pasta so much that I lose all self-control and eat until my stomach is so distended that I must stop. Wrap anything in a tortilla, and I am one happy girl. I shared my admiration for French fries, but don't even get me started on Doritos. I freakin' love Doritos! In college, I snacked on Doritos whenever I had to cram for an exam or concentrate on an assignment. I did this so often that, to this day, I still crave a salty, crunchy, cheesy snack to help me concentrate. I created a bad habit for myself, and the *perception* that I need certain foods to concentrate lingers with me today.

Have you created any bad food habits? Or maybe you haven't realized that you have developed unhealthy food habits until now. After all, habits are things we do mindlessly. Unfortunately, when we eat mindlessly, we tend to overindulge. Some of the most common acts of mindless eating are:

- Snacking while watching TV
- Grazing for something sweet before bed
- Snacking on chips because you are starving by the time you get home and just need a little something while you prepare dinner
- Having dessert after dinner because you have done this since childhood

We all have our weaknesses and unhealthy food habits. The good news is that you can still enjoy your favorite snacks and meals while integrating healthier choices or simply by cutting back on the amount of food you eat. True story. Keep reading...

I don't believe in omitting the foods you love. It is unrealistic and one of the main reasons diets fail. I would laugh at anyone who suggests I give up French fries. I have no plans to stop enjoying them, and I know you will continue to eat your favorite foods. So, let's make a pact that we will not create unrealistic plans that we do not desire to follow through with. Good? Fantastic!

I also want us to make a pact that you will be real and truthful with yourself. One of my biggest pet peeves is when a client says, *"I don't know why I can't lose weight; all I eat is salad."* I call bullshit on that excuse in nine out of ten cases because it is not always truthful. You must be honest with yourself. Do you recall me sharing this tidbit of information with you on Day 1:

...get ready to work hard, throw your ego and excuses out the window, and be prepared to get real with yourself. You will dig deep to find what is important to you, have clarity about the goals that suit you, and be

motivated to push through even when you feel like giving up. Because your health is important to you. You want to live a youthful existence. You want to live a life free of disease. **You want limitless health.**

Today, you will focus on a few things; the first one is *no more excuses.* I want you to do exactly what you set out to do when you picked up this book. I want you to live a life with limitless health by making healthy choices in the moment. We all overeat the foods we love. They are so darn good, and that's why we *love* them. So, let's find a way to love your favorite foods without feeling like you have to explain why you are eating them. I am a proud lover of French fries, and I don't make excuses for the foods I choose to eat. Today, I will share with you strategies to *mindfully* enjoy the foods you love without overindulging.

There are two things I want you to focus on: Moderation and Mindful Eating. You can enjoy the foods you love while having the not-so-healthy foods in moderation. These include foods that are high in sodium and saturated fat and contain refined carbohydrates and added sugars. You know the foods that I am talking about. In addition to eating in moderation, I want you to be mindful of your choices and how much you eat. Let's get started.

Moderation

Do you like pizza? I love pizza and have no problem eating three slices. But eating three slices will put me in a foggy headspace (Hello Day 16). Not to mention that pizza contains processed grains and, depending on the toppings, can be a source of sodium, saturated fat, and added sugar. Most sauces from a jar contain high fructose corn syrup.

I suggest enjoying one slice of pizza and a bowl of leafy greens. After enjoying the salad and slice of pizza, take a moment to determine if you are satisfied, full, or still hungry. If you are still hungry, grab a second slice of pizza. I usually do and typically feel very satisfied and content to stop eating. It's a win-win situation. You enjoy a food you love but are also making a healthy choice to eat less.

In life, we strive for balance. We also need to balance our food choices, and sometimes, balance means enjoying foods that make us happy without guilt. While I would not advise someone to eat an entire pizza, I welcome my clients to enjoy a beautiful green leafy salad with one to two slices of pizza. And eat that pizza surrounded by people who make you happy and make you laugh.

The same goes for tacos. Start with two chicken tacos loaded with veggies such as shredded cabbage, diced tomatoes, and sliced radishes. Go light on the cheese and add sliced avocado. You can also swap out the flour tortilla for a corn tortilla for fewer calories. The fiber from the veggies and healthy fat from the avocado will leave you satisfied and less likely to grab another taco. Another winning situation. You still get to enjoy delicious tacos, but you also nurture your body with fiber and healthy fat. You will walk away feeling satisfied and proud for not overdoing it.

Who doesn't love a big, juicy cheeseburger? Instead of ordering a burger for yourself, split it with someone. I split meals with my husband all the time. You may think you need your own meal, but you don't. Most portions served at restaurants provide 3-4 servings. You can still enjoy the burger and fries, but instead, eat half of what you usually do. You can also replace the fries with a healthy side dish, such as grilled veggies. If you are eating solo, ask the server to plate half of the portion and take the rest.

When it comes to pasta, order it as a side dish rather than an entree. Your main entree should be a protein, such as chicken or fish, with a delicious side of pasta or veggies. As much as I love pasta, I eat a lot less when I order it as a side.

Mindful Eating

In addition to making smart choices, keep practicing the Mindful Eating strategies you learned early on. Take your time and enjoy your meal. Be conscientious of the cues your body sends you. Remember, your brain and gut communicate, but it takes a little time to register how you feel.

Another factor I want you to consider is the perception that you need a specific food or a certain amount. For example, "I need Doritos to concentrate." In reality, I absolutely *do not* need Doritos; instead, I have created the *perception* that I need Doritos to concentrate. And these perceptions are deeply rooted in our habits. And habits are things that we do *mindlessly*.

We habitually fill our plates with food based on our perception of what and how much we need. You believe what you perceive, which can lead to unhealthy habits, such as overeating and making excuses. In addition to being truthful with yourself today, I will ask that you change your mindset and ditch old perceptions that no longer serve you.

Lastly, I want you to get real with yourself. If you struggle with how much you eat, ask yourself why. Why do you eat more than you need to? That's a difficult question with no easy answer because so many factors affect our choices. But you can answer the following:

- Can I eat less and feel content and satisfied?
- Can I be mindful about how much I eat?
- Can I eat my favorite unhealthy foods in moderation?

Absolutely! You can and will continue to enjoy the foods you love mindfully and in moderation. The best way to move forward is to modify *how* much you eat and the *perception* that you need more to feel satisfied. Here are additional tips:

Don't feel compelled to eat everything in one sitting. The next day, it will be there waiting for you as a delicious snack or lunch. In addition, when you don't overeat, you will experience the following:

- Savor the flavors of your favorite food
- Enjoy conversation with those around you
- Walk away feeling great about yourself
- Have a good night's rest
- Relish in feeling content and happy

In addition, you will consume fewer calories at each meal by simply cutting back the amount of food you eat. If you find yourself in a situation where the food is so darn good you don't want to stop eating, I have a simple solution. Brush your teeth. Remove the taste from your mouth. I know it sounds strange, but this really works.

We continue to eat when we enjoy the taste of something. When the taste dissipates, you no longer have the desire to eat. So, remove the taste! I always have a stash of disposable little toothbrushes because I am obsessed with brushing and flossing my teeth. They have a perfect little dollop of toothpaste nestled within the bristles on one end and a point on the other, similar to a toothpick. So, when you are struggling with the decision to eat a little more because the food is so darn good, grab one of these little toothbrushes instead. You can buy them at the grocery store or just about any drugstore.

For my nighttime snackers, keep healthy options in the house. Since reading Day 13, you now have fruits sitting front and center in your refrigerator, so grab an apple instead of reaching for a sweet treat. You can also try distracting yourself by going for a walk or doing a set of sit-ups.

We all know that feeling of coming home starving after a long day at work. There are a couple of choices to consider in these moments. The first thing is to eat something, but not just anything. Snack on a piece of fruit or a source of protein, such as a leftover piece of chicken, hard-boiled egg, or a handful of nuts. Don't forget that fiber makes you feel satisfied, and a small amount goes a long way.

It is also a good idea to pay attention to how much you are eating. When we are hungry, we tend to lose control of how much we eat and completely ignore any cues our body sends. The worst thing you can do is to sit down with a bag of chips. We are all guilty of being so hungry we ate the bag of chips. Instead, grab just a little and put the container away.

For example, take a *handful* of nuts, or eat *one* hard-boiled egg, or *one* tablespoon of almond butter, or *two ounces* of chicken. If it must be chips, grab a handful and put the bag away. Out of sight, out of mind. Once you have a light snack, your blood sugar levels will stabilize, and you can move on with preparing a healthy dinner.

I also urge you to reflect on what you are eating for lunch. A balanced lunch with fiber-rich foods, healthy fat, and protein will sustain you until you get home to make dinner. If you are always starving by the time you get home, it may be time to rethink your lunch choices. Choose foods that will keep you feeling full until you get home. An example for lunch is a Quinoa Bowl with quinoa, grilled chicken, black beans, roasted red peppers, feta cheese, and raw spinach drizzled with extra virgin olive oil.

Lastly, you may want to eat a small snack on the way home, such as a handful of nuts, an apple, or something left over from your lunch that day. It's just enough to keep you content until dinner is served. You know what you need to do. You know which foods make you feel good. And you know how much you should eat to feel satisfied. Choose more of that! Gone are the days of overeating. You got this, my friend.

Summary:

- You can still enjoy your favorite snacks and meals while integrating healthier choices.

- Moderation and Mindful Eating are the two things you must remember before diving into your meal head first.

- Take your time and enjoy your meal.

- Be conscientious of the cues your body sends you.

- Habits are things that we do *mindlessly*.

Achievable Actions:

- Practice Mindful Eating strategies at each meal to avoid overeating.

- Share a meal the next time you are at a restaurant.

- Brush your teeth after a meal to remove the taste of food.

Day 20

Date Night

I love date nights with my husband. I love sharing a meal with my friends while we laugh, reminisce, and solve the world's problems. I also love a quiet evening at home or taking some much-needed alone time from life's responsibilities at a cafe for lunch. Date night can be whatever it means to you. Time together, time alone, time for reflection. But one thing these options have in common is that it is a time to eat out. On average, adults eat out at restaurants about seven times per week. It's easy to do when considering breakfast, lunch, dinner, and snacks.

Eating out is fun and social, but it's also linked to overeating and poor food choices. The open-concept kitchen, the display of unbelievable desserts staring at you while waiting to be seated, and the huge menu you have to sort through that subliminally tells you to order the most fattening meal are all factors that can easily derail your intentions to eat a healthy meal. There are too many distractions, and it can be overwhelming. But it doesn't have to be if you follow a few of my favorite dining-out tips.

→ **Read the menu before you go.**

You are more likely to make unhealthy choices if you are distracted by your friends or arrive hungry. Read the menu online before you go and decide what you will order. Once you get to the restaurant, skip looking at the menu so you don't change your mind.

→ **Be the first to order.**

People tend to mimic each other subconsciously in social situations, and dining out is no exception. The choices of others can influence eating behaviors at the table. To avoid the "Oh, that sounds good. I will have the same," place your order first.

→ **Don't show up hungry.**

Have a healthy snack before you arrive so that you are not starving. Again, we tend to make unhealthy choices when we are hungry. I know I don't think clearly when I am starving, and I can get downright hangry. So, have an apple or a pear on your way to the restaurant. A healthy snack beforehand will prevent *hangry* ordering.

→ **Avoid unnecessary calories.**

Look for food that is steamed, grilled, roasted, or poached. In general, these cooking methods equate to fewer calories. Pan-fried, fried, crispy, crunchy, or sautéed will usually contain more fat and calories.

→ **Put it on the side.**

Ask for sauces, condiments, and salad dressings on the side. Sauces and dressings can add a lot of extra fat and calories to a dish, so ask for your sauce on the side to avoid excess calories. Keeping it separate will help you control how much you eat.

→ **Start with a soup or salad.**

The fiber from salad will make you feel full so you don't overeat during the meal. Having soup before can reduce your total calorie intake by 20%. Avoid soups made with cream if you are lactose intolerant or want to watch your caloric intake.

→ **Order an appetizer as your meal.**

Restaurants are notorious for serving large portions. Most meals include 2-3 portions, so order one or two appetizers instead of a main course.

→ **Share a meal.**

Sharing a meal is a simple way to reduce calories and prevent overeating. I mentioned yesterday that I share meals with my husband all the time. If you don't have someone to share with, ask the waiter for a half-portion or to wrap up half your meal to take home.

→ **Swap the side dish.**

You can always swap the side dish for a healthier alternative. I love fries, but more often than not, I switch them out for a side salad or grilled veggies. You'll boost your fiber intake and cut excess calories.

→ **Skip the chips and salsa.**

Okay, this is a hard one. We all love the bowl of chips and salsa served at Mexican restaurants. Or the basket filled with warm bread and salted butter. I know, I know. It's hard to resist. But you can do it. Just say no. If you must, put some on a plate and ask the server to remove the remaining so you don't overindulge.

→ **Drink water.**

Replacing sugar-sweetened drinks such as soda or juice with water can help reduce your intake of calories and added sugar. One soda is about 150-240 calories, depending on the size.

→ **Drink wisely.**

The calories can add up quickly if you are enjoying cocktails with dinner. For example, a generous glass of red wine can add around 280 calories to your meal. Unfortunately, that's the same as a Snickers bar. If you want to enjoy a cocktail, cut back on the extra calories by ordering a smaller pour, or choose a mixed drink with sparkling water/soda, such as vodka and soda with lime.

→ **Practice Mindful Eating.**

As you can tell, I am a fan of this technique. Because it works! Take your time and eat mindfully. We tend to overeat in social settings because we are distracted. You are more likely to overeat if dining with a group because you are not paying attention to how much you eat or how you feel. Enjoy your company, but take time to listen to your body.

→ **Enjoy a cup of Joe instead of dessert.**

Order a cup of coffee and skip the dessert. You will cut out a lot of calories and added sugar.

→ **Enjoy yourself.**

Don't complicate dining out. If you are eating healthy foods and making smart choices most of the time, go ahead and treat yourself. An occasional indulgence can be good for the soul.

When it comes to eating in general, be concerned with what you do most of the time rather than what you do sometimes. If you eat healthy most of the time, don't sweat the small stuff of what you do some of the time. For example, I eat healthy during the week by cooking at home. On the weekends, I enjoy a good date night with my hubby or a night out with friends at an amazing restaurant. Remind yourself that it's okay to overeat or dive into your favorite comfort foods occasionally.

In addition to today's tips, use yesterday's advice to help plan your next romantic date with your significant other. How often have you and your partner crawled into bed after eating out because you ate too much or something that didn't agree with you? Who wants to be gassy and bloated when you are trying to get the sparks flying? Overeating or ordering the wrong foods will send you straight to bed without any sexy time with your partner. Instead, share an appetizer, split a salad, and order one entrée. You can always order more if you are still hungry. In most cases, there will be plenty of food, and you will leave the restaurant feeling good and ready to take your date to the next level.

I suggest taking your time in between each course. No rule says you have to order everything at once. Do you notice that once the food starts coming, it's one dish after another, and it turns into a marathon race to the food finish line? Instead, order an appetizer and enjoy it. Then, order a soup or salad. Taking time between the courses allows you to listen to the internal hunger cues and if you truly need to order more food.

Enjoy your date night!

Summary:

- On average, adults eat out about seven times per week.

- Eating out is fun and social, but it's also linked to overeating and poor food choices.

- Be concerned with what you do most of the time rather than what you do sometimes.

- Remind yourself that it's okay to overeat or dive into your favorite comfort foods occasionally.

- Take your time in between each course. No rule says you have to order everything at once.

Achievable Actions:

- Apply at least two of today's tips the next time you eat out.

- Order one course at a time rather than ordering everything at once to allow time to determine if you are still hungry.

- Incorporate at least two tips from yesterday to avoid overeating.

Day 21

Create the Life You Want to Live

Over the past 20 days, you have tried new things, overcome fears, and pushed yourself past your limits. One thing I want you to take away from this book is not to allow limitations, challenges, or tragedies to define your abilities. Take the time to be honest with yourself, sit with your discomfort, and take action to change. This is how you open the door to healing and self-efficacy.

If a strategy in this book didn't work for you, but you really wanted it to, consider changing your approach. Sometimes, you have to approach things differently to make it work. No one says you can't tweak the strategies I have shared with you. There are no rules here. This is not a fad diet book; I am not the nutrition police. Utilize the strategies that work for you, absorb the information in this book, and determine the best action plan for *you*.

Living a healthy life is not difficult. As you progress in your health journey, be prudent of people who complicate health and nutrition. Influencers and health coaches will often obscure the facts, either because they don't truly understand the advice they are offering, or they are trying to sound smart to influence you to purchase a product, supplement, or fad diet. If something seems too good to be true, it likely is. And if something is too complicated, move on! Don't complicate your life with a nutrition plan that doesn't make sense or serve you.

Nutrition science is clear, but dietary advice changes as new scientific evidence emerges. Unfortunately, this can lead to consumer confusion. I have three degrees in nutrition, but I never stop learning. My job is to decipher the scientific evidence to provide actionable advice to others. The good news is that you don't need to know the complicated science. Instead, I want you to focus on the basic needs that support long-term health.

This book has provided you with the basics to live a healthy lifestyle. These basics allow you to try new foods, strategies, and confidently make healthy choices. A healthy lifestyle can be quite simple. And I have a secret to share with you. You will never achieve "well-being." Well-being is an infinite journey that you will continually work on. A healthy lifestyle is limitless.

From this day forward, I want you to stop placing unrealistic expectations and outlandish goals upon yourself. Don't strive to achieve goals that are unrealistic and unattainable. It's not that you *can't* achieve these goals. You can do anything you want. But you won't accomplish goals that don't serve a purpose in *your* life. Too often, we try to achieve something that serves someone else: your boss, significant other, your friends. When you stop achieving the goals of others, you will free yourself to do things that truly matter and make a difference.

In addition to learning new strategies, you have made many healthy choices. Healthy choices for *you*. The more you do this, the easier it is to create healthy habits. And the best is yet to come. Eventually, these new habits will become second nature, and you will do them without thinking about it. It will be as easy as brushing your teeth in the morning.

Throughout the book, I focus on nutrition and a healthy diet. It is important to recognize that your diet is not only what you eat. It's what you listen to, what you watch, what you read, and the people that you surround yourself with. It is important to be mindful of the information you absorb, as it can affect your body emotionally, physically, and spiritually. This is true with any change you want to embrace, not just your diet.

By now, you are likely crushing several new habits. I'm proud of you for trying new things and for being good to yourself. You may have even come up with your own achievable actions. When you do something good for yourself, you will continue to find new, healthy actions that make you feel even better about yourself. You may find that you are pushing yourself beyond your limitations. In addition, I hope you are doing so well that you have influenced others to make healthy choices, too.

Before we end this day, I have a few questions.

- What did it take to establish a new routine?
- What worked for you?
- What didn't work for you, and how did you overcome challenges?
- Have you yet to begin making any changes?

If you haven't made any changes, ask yourself why. What obstacle created a barrier for you? What stood in your way? To get around something, sometimes you have to go through it. Meaning you have to persevere and do the work. But to do the work, you have to want it badly enough. And I know that you do want it, or else you would not have spent time reading this book.

If you chose to read the book before attempting to adopt any new healthy behaviors, I ask that you do just one achievable action today. Please answer the following questions:

- Who do you see yourself becoming if you can achieve your ultimate health goal?
- How badly do you want it?
- What obstacles stand in your way, and how can you move past them?
- What will happen if you do not achieve your goal?

Here are a few scenarios for the above questions:

Who do you see yourself becoming if you can achieve your ultimate health goal?

- I see myself as a healthier version of myself, walking into a room with the confidence of a lion.
- I am that person who is physically active every day, and I love pushing myself to new heights.
- I am a parent who leads by example.
- I am walking on the beach in a bathing suit, and I feel great.

How badly do you want it?

- I want to achieve these healthy goals more than anything, and I will not let anything stand in my way.
- I owe it to myself to take the necessary steps to be healthy, vital, and feel young.
- I want it so badly that I will not only motivate myself, but I will lead by example for my family and friends.

What obstacles stand in your way, and how can you move past them?

- I love food. I enjoy eating, but it is hard to stop, so I will only prepare enough so that I will not overindulge.
- I will eat mindfully and listen to the internal hunger cues telling me to stop eating.

What will happen if you do not achieve your goal?

- I will not like the person that I am.
- I will live with limitations.
- I will choose to eat foods that do not nourish my body.
- I will not be physically fit.
- I will be okay with who I am in this moment.

It is great to make healthy changes. It is okay to remain as you are if you are not ready. Either way, make a choice and be happy with your choice. Make choices that fulfill you and bring you joy. But if you are struggling with where to begin, my advice is just to begin. You have to start somewhere.

The hardest thing about losing weight or working out is starting. Change is hard at first, messy in the middle, but glorious at the end. Deep down, you know what you need to do, and you know that you need to start. And let me tell you, staying motivated is its own separate challenge. But, if you can get past those hurdles and do the things that don't excite you, I promise there will come a time when jumping the hurdles is the best part of your day. Truly, you will love working out. You will love how you feel after eating nourishing meals every day. You will feel so good you will share your struggles and triumphs with others. I promise you, this will happen. You only need to make the choice, in the moment, to live with limitless health.

Acknowledgments

I would like to express my sincere gratitude to the following individuals who have played a significant role in the creation and publication of this book:

I want to extend a special note of gratitude to my husband, Rob, who has been my anchor throughout the journey of writing this book. Thank you for always being there, for your unwavering belief in my work, and for the countless sacrifices you've made to see this book come to life. Your support, encouragement, and understanding have been my constant inspiration. Your love has sustained me through the challenges and celebrated with me in the triumphs. This book is as much yours as it is mine. Thank you for being there in every chapter of our story. I love you, handsome.

My family, thank you for being the foundation of my life and for sharing this incredible journey with me.

My dear friends, who provided encouragement and motivation when I needed it most.

My editor and publishing team, for their invaluable guidance and expertise in making this book a reality.

My readers, without whom this book would have no purpose. I want to express my deepest appreciation to each and every one of you who has picked up this book, turned its pages, and allowed its words to become a part of your life.

With heartfelt gratitude,

Tammy

About the Author

Tammy Fogarty is a passionate and dedicated registered dietitian and nutritionist who's committed to helping everyone lead their healthiest life. With more than 23 years experience, her commitment to evidence-based practice has helped hundreds of clients and readers reach their health goals.

Tammy earned her undergraduate and graduate degrees, including a Ph.D. in Nutrition and Dietetics from Florida International University. Throughout her career, she has held roles in clinical and community nutrition and currently runs her private practice, About Thyme Nutrition. Tammy helps her clients with multiple nutritional needs, from managing chronic conditions to achieving weight loss. She also provides online nutrition programs available at www.tammyfogarty.com.

Tammy practices yoga daily and earned her 200-hour teaching certification. In 2018, she conducted a research study providing a yoga and nutrition intervention to breast cancer survivors to promote quality of life and improve dietary intake.

Tammy lives in South Florida with her husband, Rob, and their two dogs, Molly and Mugsy, where they enjoy their time cooking, boating, staying fit, and traveling. Tammy and Rob love spending time with friends and their growing family, including Rob's two children David and Lisa, daughter-in-law Alex, and two beautiful grandchildren, Emma and Johnny.